Case Studies in Neurological Rehabilitation

nerever you are

onditions:

ee our details below.

ea by

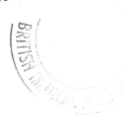

D1435127

Case Studies in Neurological Rehabilitation

Tarek A.-Z. K. Gaber

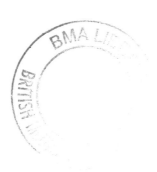

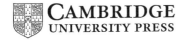

CAMBRIDGE
UNIVERSITY PRESS

CAMBRIDGE UNIVERSITY PRESS
Cambridge, New York, Melbourne, Madrid, Cape Town, Singapore, São Paulo, Delhi

Cambridge University Press
The Edinburgh Building, Cambridge CB2 8RU, UK

Published in the United States of America by Cambridge University Press, New York

www.cambridge.org
Information on this title: www.cambridge.org/9780521697163

First published 2008

Printed in the United Kingdom at the University Press, Cambridge

A catalogue record for this publication is available from the British Library

ISBN 978-0-521-69716-3 paperback

Contents

Preface   *page* ix

Part I Clinical rehabilitation

1   The rehabilitation consultation   **3**

2   The rehabilitation unit   **6**

Part II Case studies

3   **Medical issues in brain injury rehabilitation**   **11**

Post-traumatic seizures   12
Agitation following herpes simplex encephalitis   15
Hypopituitarism following brain injury   17
Anxiety following head injury   20
Hydrocephalus following subarachnoid haemorrhage   23
Autonomic impairment following brain injury   26
Locked-in syndrome   29
Pharmacological management of attention impairment   32
Rehabilitation of pontine myelinolysis   34
Assessment of frontal lobe function   37
An aggressive patient   41

4   **Progressive neurological disorders**   **44**

Ataxia in multiple sclerosis   45
Psychiatric manifestations in Huntington's disease   48
The adult patient with Duchenne muscular dystrophy   51
Recurrent aspiration in a patient with Parkinson's disease   53

5   **Medical complications of immobility**   **57**

Thromboembolism   57
Osteoporosis   61
Pressure sores   64
Heterotopic ossification   67

6 Orthotics in neurological rehabilitation   **70**
Secondary scoliosis   71
Post polio syndrome   74
Charcot arthropathy   78

7 Ethical and medicolegal controversies   **82**
A wandering patient   83
Rehabilitation of the patient from an ethnic minority   85
Service provision for chronic fatigue syndrome   87

8 Chronic pain   **91**
Central pain syndrome   91
Complex regional pain syndrome   94
Shoulder pain following stroke   97

9 Medically unexplained disorders   **101**
Conversion syndrome   101
Somatisation in multiple sclerosis   104
Complementary and alternative medicine   107

10 Spasticity management   **110**
Management of spastic equinovarus deformity   110
Management of generalised severe spasticity   113

11 Ventilatory support in rehabilitation   **117**
Artificial ventilation in Guillain–Barré syndrome   117
Diaphragmatic paralysis   120

12 Sphincteric dysfunction   **123**
Botulinum toxin for neuropathic bladder   123
Bowel dysfunction following spinal injury   126

13 Communication disabilities   **130**
Expressive aphasia   130
Jargon aphasia   134
Hypokinetic dysarthria   136

14 Sensory disability   **139**
Cortical blindness   139
Visual spatial neglect   142

15 Prescriptions for independence   **146**
Exercise prescription   146
Vocational rehabilitation   149
Driving assessment   152

Part III Exercises in neurological rehabilitation

Multiple choice questions   157

Multiple choice answers   174

Index   181

Preface

During my specialist rehabilitation medicine training in Cambridge, I tried to find a suitable text to refer to when dealing with the usual mix of cases seen in a typical neurological rehabilitation service. I found many excellent large reference textbooks and also a few pocket books with a wealth of information. However, the popular books were either neurological texts concentrating mainly on neurological disorders as a primarily diagnostic challenge or general rehabilitation texts with a generalist approach and lacking the boldness of the standard medical texts in suggesting management plans from a medical perspective.

I wanted two main things: firstly, to know the medical management of the cases I saw and secondly to have an overview of the management of other impairments usually dealt with by other members of the team, such as psychological, physical or communication disabilities.

This book is trying to address such common issues. It is not intended as a comprehensive text covering all or even most of the common scenarios seen in a neurological rehabilitation setting; however, I hope that it will cover many common but difficult issues. The book takes the approach of presenting material as case histories. The case itself does not usually present a diagnostic problem but it is intended to set the scene for a discussion of a complex neurological rehabilitation issue. My view is that rehabilitation medicine lends itself to this kind of approach, and I have tried to make the cases as non-specific as possible to enable the commentary to address more general issues, probably adopting the mantra of the UK television programme *Panorama (BBC): behind the news there is a story and behind the story there is an issue.* So this book's philosophy can be, *behind the case there is a story and behind the story there is an issue*

The book concludes with 50 Multiple choice questions. I have used this approach to present important clinical scenarios that were not covered in the case commentaries. The style of the questions is not dissimilar to that used in some of the board examinations in Europe and North America. Therefore, I hope that examination candidates will find the questions useful.

This book is intended mainly for trainees and specialists in neurology and rehabilitation medicine. However, I hope that all the members of the neurological rehabilitation team will find the material useful. I have tried to present the medical material in an uncomplicated way to allow non-medically trained clinicians to follow the arguments with ease.

I have avoided long references lists after each case as I feel that at this time, and thanks to the Internet and sites such as *Pubmed* and *Google Scholar*, the most recent literature is available online for everyone; probably many ground-breaking papers will have been released by the time the book is published. I have only suggested two or three references that might complement the information the cases presented.

It is not easy to find randomised controlled trials guiding issues such as management of frontal lobe cognitive impairments or rehabilitation of patients with pontine myelinolysis. Therefore, the advice given is based on both the literature available and the experiences of the author and the contributors of cases and ideas, who all practise in the UK. I hope that the book will be valuable for clinicians dealing with neurologically impaired people everywhere around the world, as I have tried to avoid reference to any UK laws as much as possible. In a few cases, such laws are mentioned, for example the sections on mental health, I feel that the arguments can be generalised to most societies and populations.

I would like to thank my colleagues and friends Ashraf Azer, Janet Blakeley, Barry Clift, Salem Madi, Carolyn McAllister, Russell Sheldrick and Sarah Wilkinson for contributing several cases and ideas for the book. I would like also to thank Jai Kulkarni and Sue Comish for reviewing the text, my wife Solveig for her help with the manuscript preparation and my publisher Richard Marley for all his help throughout the project.

Part I

Clinical rehabilitation

The rehabilitation consultation

In a rehabilitation setting, the medical/neurological clinic should be more than a standard consultation aiming at diagnosis and medical management of the clinical condition. Beside this core function, the clinic appointment should be a chance for the patient to be assessed in the most comprehensive way. Most neurologically disabled patients will have complex problems such as medical, physical, psychological, mental health, communication, swallowing, sphincteric, tissue viability, equipment, social, financial, and probably more obscure but nonetheless crucial issues. Most members of the rehabilitation team concentrate on the management of the problem relevant to them, with relatively limited ability to appreciate the impact other disabilities are having and the complex way they can interact together to generate a management problem. For example, a patient with multiple sclerosis who presents with falls may also have a bladder problem, with urgency and frequency of micturition, plus a visual impairment and, consequently, may fall while rushing to the toilet.

The rehabilitation clinic should act as the clinical setting to look at the patient with a wide perspective. Rehabilitation physicians should have the ability to evaluate all the relevant pieces of the puzzle and to use their knowledge of the basic practice principles of other therapists/clinicians in order to 'plug' the patient into the appropriate services and to review their progress and ensure that goals are achieved.

Rehabilitation physicians should always work in direct contact with the members of their team. This will avoid lengthy paper trails, misunderstandings and, most importantly, disagreements regarding how realistic some goals are. Some clinicians adopt the model of *joint clinics*, where the patients are seen by the physician and one or two relevant members of the team. I personally find this model extremely helpful and a very efficient way to use time and resources. A patient with a gait impairment resulting from a combination of weakness and spasticity can be seen by the physician and the physiotherapist. A management plan can be formulated with the agreement of the clinicians and the patient. If an intervention such as botulinum toxin injections is suggested, decisions about which muscles to be injected and postinjection physiotherapy can be arranged on the spot without delays or misunderstandings.

This model of service provision is very difficult to implement within the context of a standard hospital clinic service where general practitioner (GP) referrals are automatically placed into vacant clinic slots. From my experience, GP referrals are not the major source of patients in a rehabilitation clinic. It is unfair to ask GPs to determine which disciplines in the rehabilitation team the patient should see and whether medical input will be needed or not. A more appropriate approach is to encourage GPs to refer their patients to the neurological rehabilitation team and then leave it for the members of the team to determine which clinicians should see the patient. The majority of patients will probably not need a specialist medical rehabilitation input and many of them will be under neurological consultants for their primary diagnosis. An experienced member of the team can do the initial patient's assessment and then can refer to the rehabilitation medical clinic accordingly. Specific groups of patients stand out as the most in need of such a comprehensive approach as they often present with complex management issues. Brain injury, whether traumatic or secondary to other causes such as encephalitis, often presents with complex physical and cognitive issues needing a holistic approach to their management. Patients with spinal injuries are usually young with many psychological, social and vocational issues that need to be addressed in conjunction with their primary physical problems. Other conditions such as multiple sclerosis may also benefit from such an approach. Patients with cerebral palsy or spina bifida will probably need annual reviews as many of the problems they face are subtle with an insidious onset and have the potential to lead to long-term major problems such as chronic pain syndromes or renal failure. A specialist review will increase the early detection of such problems.

Management of medically unexplained conditions such as conversion syndrome, pseudo-seizures or chronic fatigue syndrome should ideally be the responsibility of a neurological rehabilitation service. Such disorders are difficult, complex and need a well-coordinated rehabilitation effort, with one or two key clinicians acting as a source of motivation, support and information for the patients.

One of the advantages of such a model of service provision is that it reduces the need for regular medical follow-ups, freeing spaces for new patients and for patients with active medical issues. Once the initial joint medical assessment is concluded, a comprehensive action plan can be formulated and copies distributed to clinicians involved and to the patient and/or carers. This management plan can act as a template for reviews in the near future, with the therapist most involved with the patient reviewing the goals. The patient can then be brought back into the medical clinic once a new medical issue or a complex problem that warrants a medical review arises.

Many patients will be too immobile to be able to come to the clinic and will need a domiciliary visit. Again a joint visit with the therapist can achieve much more than a visit by the physician addressing only medical issues. The visit will be a good opportunity to increase the team's appreciation of the psychosocial context of the patient's presentations so that appropriate management steps can be taken.

2

The rehabilitation unit

Most neurological rehabilitation units admit patients following acute neurological damage such as brain injury, spinal injury or stroke. The standard practice is to admit patients once they are medically stable, assuming that the patient has good potential for rehabilitation. The necessity of medical stability as an essential requirement for accepting the patient for an inpatient rehabilitation programme is not only to ensure that the patient is able to tolerate therapy but also because of the relative inexperience of the rehabilitation team in dealing with acute and active complex medical issues. Rehabilitation units will certainly differ in their staffing, location and philosophy, with some units geared more towards accepting patients early on after the neurological insult and others accepting patients in after the acute stage. In the acute stage following a neurological insult such as a traumatic head injury, encephalitis or subarachnoid haemorrhage, rehabilitation needs are unique and involve mainly issues such as tracheostomy management, maintaining the range of movements in joints, management of early seizures or managing cognitive or behavioural impairments during the period of post-traumatic amnesia. It is essential that a service dealing with this stage has the expertise to manage such acute stage problems, sufficient staff, an intensity of medical input and a location that ensures immediate access to specialist medical and surgical support. A unit accepting patients at a later stage of their rehabilitation may need less intense medical input but should have different facilities such as designated large therapy areas, occupational therapy kitchens or small flats for independent living to evaluate patients before discharge.

In Greater Manchester, the neurological rehabilitation services have been configured and organised regionally to ensure that the patients' rehabilitation needs in the acute, post-acute and chronic stages are met. The regional neuroscience unit is based at Hope Hospital, Salford with an acute neurological rehabilitation ward being a part of the neuroscience department. This ward accepts patients in the acute stage following any neurological insult such as brain injury or after neurosurgical interventions for conditions such as subdural haematomas, subarachnoid haemorrhage or brain tumour. The acute rehabilitation unit serves three million Greater Manchester residents. Once the patient is neurologically stable, he/she can be transferred to one of four intermediate rehabilitation units located in different centres: Wigan, Stockport, Rochdale and central Manchester. The acute rehabilitation unit and the four intermediate rehabilitation units function as a *service network* for issues such as clinical governance, outcome measures and lobbying for resources. Despite the persistence of inequalities in access to some aspects of community rehabilitation and in transfer waiting times, this model of service has helped greatly in the provision of neurological rehabilitation services for Greater Manchester residents irrespective of the area they live in (postcode).

Patients with chronic neurological disabilities such as multiple sclerosis or Parkinson's disease form an important clientele to the neurological rehabilitation units. Such patients are usually admitted either straight from home or they may be transferred from an acute ward following an acute admission to manage problems such as bony fractures, infections or general deterioration of functional abilities through natural progression of the primary neurological condition. The intermediate neurological rehabilitation units usually have a case mix of patients with post-acute or chronic neurological rehabilitation conditions.

The basic philosophy and ideas of rehabilitation should be introduced to the patient in the early period following admission. Concepts such as goal setting, supporting the patient to achieve independence, instead of simply providing basic care, and interdisciplinary work of the staff are all important and the patient should be able to grasp these concepts if he/she is going to be able to participate fully into the rehabilitation programme. For example, a patient accepting the philosophy of interdisciplinary work will appreciate that help during washing and dressing, transfers or meals are all integral to the physiotherapy and occupational therapy sessions; consequently, he/she would not feel disappointed about the length and frequency of the formal therapy sessions. Explicit goal setting may help another patient to appreciate the progress that he/she is making and can also help him/her to focus on a particular functional task even during evenings and weekends when formal therapy is not usually available.

The length of stay for patients can be from a few weeks to several months; consequently it is not uncommon for patients to feel low in mood and homesick. Early assessment for home leave can help to alleviate these feelings. We have also found that the role of an *activity coordinator* can greatly enhance the patients' enjoyment and improve their mood. The activity coordinator usually spends long hours with the patients and is in a very good position to pick up any subtle social, behavioural or mood problems, such as anxiety. Our activity coordinator is a valuable member of the team and her contributions in the team meetings and case conferences are invaluable as they increase the team member's insight regarding their patients' mood or other important issues. The activity coordinator can also help in the difficult times immediately following discharge by providing an outreach service to reduce the potential for social isolation for vulnerable patients.

For many patients, discharge from the rehabilitation unit is synonymous with the conclusion of their rehabilitation and the frightening prospect of a life with their residual disability with only minimal efforts for further rehabilitation. The community rehabilitation programme should be discussed fully with the patient to reassure him/her about the future. A few patients will refuse to accept discharge as they feel that they are still able to achieve further improvement with inpatient therapy. One of the ways to demonstrate to the patient the lack of progress is to set one or two modest goals with a specific time frame to achieve these goals. Failure to achieve the goals in the agreed period can demonstrate to the patient the difficulty of achieving further improvement. For example, a patient failing to achieve good sitting balance will be unable to achieve further goals relevant to physical transfers.

Other patients might be desperate to be discharged but the plans for discharge are delayed because of the unsuitability of their discharge destination. Such patients should be identified as soon as possible and plans made for home adaptations or provision of equipment. The issues relevant to discharge should be a fixed item in the case conference agenda, with the members of the rehabilitation team using their expertise to predict the functional abilities of the patient by the time of discharge and to set the wheels in motion for a discharge plan as soon as possible.

Part II

Case studies

3

Medical issues in brain injury rehabilitation

Because of its high incidence in the young population, traumatic brain injury has become one of the major challenges from a public health perspective. The overwhelming majority of the more than one million patients attending accident and emergency departments in Britain each year will have mild head injury and will suffer mild and transient symptoms with no long-term complications. However, a minority of those patients with mild head injury will suffer significant chronic cognitive impairments that will impact on their social and/or vocational functions. Glasgow Coma Scale assessment plus the period of post-traumatic amnesia have traditionally been used to determine the severity of the head injury; amnesia of less than an hour indicating a mild head injury, for 1–24 hours indicating moderate injury and for more than 24 hours indicating severe head injury.

Clinically, neither severity of the head injury nor brain scan findings are able to indicate unequivocally the long-term prognosis, with many patients with a mild head injury and normal scans going on to develop significant cognitive or behavioural disabilities that will impact on their social and/or vocational functions while full recovery following a moderately severe head injury is occasionally seen.

Different service models have been suggested to try to screen patients with mild brain injury for cognitive impairments, with accident and emergency follow-up clinics for mild brain injury being commonly used. Accident and emergency departments provide patients with written information about symptoms of post-concussion syndrome and advise them to contact their GP if the symptoms persist.

Most brain injury rehabilitation services are geared towards the severely injured patients, as they clearly require a multidisciplinary approach for management to cater for their complex physical, cognitive and behavioural problems. Several medical complications are commonly seen in patients with brain injury. Recognition and appropriate management of these complications is an important element in the overall rehabilitation effort.

Post-traumatic seizures

A 22-year-old man sustained a severe head injury judging by post-traumatic amnesia for 10 days and a Glasgow Coma Score of 4/15 in the first 24 hours after injury. The head computed tomographic (CT) scan showed evidence of frontal contusion and the patient was managed conservatively. The patient had two generalised seizures, the first immediately after the accident while awaiting the ambulance and the second two days later. He was managed with phenytoin 300 mg daily. The patient progressed very well with his rehabilitation and two months later discontinuation of phenytoin was discussed with him and his family.

Comments

Up to 10% of patients with severe head injuries suffer from post-traumatic seizures. Patients with skull fractures, intracranial haematomas and prolonged periods of unconsciousness are particularly vulnerable. Patients with mild-to-moderate head injury will also have an increased risk of seizures. However, the risk is less than 1% for such patients.

Acute post-traumatic seizures are defined as seizure activities occurring within the first week following the head injury. Such seizures are quite harmful and, therefore, aggressive management including attempts at prevention is mandatory. Acute seizures may cause further brain damage through several mechanisms, including increased brain metabolism, increased hazardous inflammatory transmitters, including free radicals, and direct mechanical cellular damage. Phenytoin has been traditionally used to manage seizures in the acute stage. Despite the availability of several newer antiepileptic drugs with a relatively safer profile, phenytoin has several unique properties that are advantageous during such a critical period. It can be administered intravenously, thus providing an almost immediate therapeutic effect. Following that initial dose, full oral dosage can be administered without the need to build up the dose slowly. Phenytoin has also been shown to possess neuroprotective properties in animal models, most probably through its sodium channel-blocking action.

The popularity of phenytoin as an antiepileptic in the acute stages of head injury makes it very common for rehabilitation physicians to see their patients with head injuries already taking it when admitted to the rehabilitation units. Rehabilitation physicians are often concerned about the sedative side effects of phenytoin as it may accentuate the patient's cognitive difficulties. The decision either to continue or to stop phenytoin will be mainly based on the need for prophylactic antiepileptic therapy to prevent late seizures.

Late post-traumatic seizures are believed to have a unique pathogenesis, which makes this an almost completely distinct condition from the acute seizures. The risk of late seizures is highest in the first two years following the acute head injury. Following that, the risk progressively reduces with time. Despite the fact that the occurrence of acute seizures will increase the risk of late seizures, the link is not strong enough to justify long-term antiepileptic therapy in most cases. Many trials have examined the use of antiepileptic drugs to reduce the risk of late seizures. Systematic reviews of these trials were conclusive. There is no evidence that post-acute anti-epileptic drugs reduce disability, mortality or risk of the development of late seizures.

The risk and rational of antiepileptic drug use should be discussed with the patient and the family in detail, and discontinuation should be strongly recommended. A few patients will insist on continuation of antiepileptic medications, especially those whose livelihoods are dependent on driving as they are usually horrified by the prospect of a single seizure disqualifying them from driving for at least a year. A new generation antiepileptic drug such as valproate, carbamazepine or lamotrigine should be offered to such patients as the safety profiles of these drugs are much better than phenytoin. The new drug should be introduced first, building up the dose slowly. When the lower end of the therapeutic range is reached, phenytoin should be withdrawn slowly. If the patient starts to develop seizures while on that regimen, the new drug dose should be increased in the usual way.

Sufficient time should be spent explaining to patients the usual triggers of seizures, mainly alcohol, dehydration, lack of sleep and stress. Alcohol is a particularly important precipitating factor as patients find it difficult to associate excessive alcohol intake with seizures. Alcohol is a neurological depressant and a few patients experience improvement of their recurrent simple partial fits (e.g. hand shakes) while drinking alcohol as it generally suppresses the brain. As the patient continues to drink they become dehydrated, leading to the classic hangover the following morning. This brain cellular dehydration is the most potent trigger for seizures. Consequently, a heavy drinking session in an evening can lead to seizures the following morning. This mechanism should be explained to the patients together with a strong recommendation to avoid alcohol. If the patients are keen to continue drinking, they should be advised to take small quantities with adequate water at the same time to avoid dehydration. Avoidance of dehydration is very important in general, especially in hot weather or with minor vomiting or diarrhoeal illnesses.

Diagnosis of simple partial, complex partial, or generalised fits is usually straightforward. A few patients will present with non-specific episodes, which will be difficult to categorise. Such patients should be referred for specialist studies such as 24 hour electroencephalography (EEG). Treatment should not be prescribed empirically as a diagnosis of epilepsy will have serious implications for the patient both socially and vocationally, and all efforts should be made to establish the diagnosis in the most confident and robust way.

Many patients present with simple partial seizures, which can generalise or develop into complex partial seizures. Simple partial seizures may present as a motor phenomenon (e.g. arm or leg shakes), a sensory phenomenon (e.g. sudden unilateral pain or paraesthesia) or as a temporal lobe phenomenon (e.g. auras such as stomach discomfort, feeling of sudden dread or a strange smell). When asked, many patients are not bothered if the partial seizures do not generalise or if they do not develop into complex seizures affecting their consciousness state. An adequate dose of an antiepileptic drug may help to prevent secondary generalisation or complex partial seizures but the partial seizures may persist. Patients should appreciate that partial seizures are *seizures*, with all the vocational and medicolegal implications associated with seizures (e.g. for driving). Complete control of all types of seizure should be the ultimate goal of a successful epilepsy management plan.

If complete abolishment of partial seizures proves difficult, either because they are refractory or because very high doses of several antiepileptic drugs are needed and lead to several side effects, clinicians can resort to a different strategy, trying to prevent the secondary generalisation or the development of complex partial seizures. These are the forms of epilepsy usually dreaded by the patients as they may lead to serious accidents such as burns or falls. Rapidly acting benzodiazepines such as clobazam or midazolam can be a very useful addition to the standard antiepileptic regimen the patient is taking regularly. Many patients will experience partial seizures for minutes or hours before the seizures generalise. Patients could be advised to take oral clobazam, intranasal midazolam or rectal diazepam as soon as they feel the first simple partial seizure, aiming for a rapid effect of the benzodiazepine. This approach should help in stopping the partial seizures or at least reducing the risk of secondary generalisation.

Further reading

Schierhout, G., Roberts, I. (2001). Anti-epileptic drugs for preventing seizures following acute traumatic brain injury. *Cochran Database Sys Rev* **4**, CD000173.

Tamkin, N. R. (2001). Antiepileptogenesis and seizure prevention trials with antiepileptic drugs: meta-analysis of controlled trials. *Epilepsia* **4**, 515–524.

Agitation following herpes simplex encephalitis

A 48-year-old woman presented with sudden confusion and fever. The diagnosis of herpes simplex encephalitis (HSE) was confirmed with a positive polymerase chain reaction test for herpes simplex virus in cerebrospinal fluid (CSF). Antiviral treatment with aciclovir was commenced and continued for two weeks. Within a few weeks, the patient made almost full physical recovery. However, she continued to have several cognitive and behavioural problems. The patient was hostile and confused, with episodes of extreme behaviour such as swearing and violent behaviour. The patient failed to respond to different antipsychotic and antidepressant medications.

A few months later, magnetic resonance imaging (MRI) showed encephalomalacia of the right temporal lobe consistent with previous HSE. An EEG was normal. In further evaluation, the nursing staff reported that the patient was generally confused but there were distinctive episodes where she would stare and then display abusive and disruptive behaviour for periods of up to 30 minutes once or twice a day.

Comments

Herpes simplex virus (HSV) is the commonest cause of sporadic encephalitis in humans. Without treatment, mortality is over 70%, with less than 3% of the patients affected returning to normal function. Aciclovir not only reduces the mortality rate to around 20%, it also has a profound effect on the development of long-term complications, especially neuropsychiatric impairments and personality changes. Before aciclovir administration became standard practice, up to 60% of survivors had long-term behavioural and cognitive problems. Recent research reports only about a 20% incidence of patients having difficulties with social or vocational activities two years after the onset of HSE.

About 90% of HSE is caused by type 1 (HSV-1). This virus usually affects healthy adults, causing a necrotising inflammatory process that eventually localises and mainly affects the frontotemporal lobes in an asymmetrical fashion. Type 2 virus affects those with an inadequate immune system, including neonates and immunocompromised patients. It has a more diffuse pathology and generally worse prognosis.

Psychiatric problems following HSE are the main cause of long-term disability in these patients. Cognitive and psychiatric problems are usually already in place in the acute stage and further deterioration or relapses are uncommon especially if aciclovir therapy was initiated early. The cognitive problems are often subtle and a normal Mini-Mental Test Score would not exclude them. Many patients will have mild cognitive impairment, which in conjunction with the psychiatric deficits can have a profound effect on the patient's vocational prospects and social integration.

Occurrence of HSE is the leading cause of refractory status epilepticus. More than 60% of HSE patients will have seizures in the acute stage. However, only 20% of them will have long-term epileptic activities. As the temporal area is the usual source of the seizure activities, epileptic activities in some patients will present as episodic behavioural disturbances. While, EEG can be a useful tool to establish the source and type of the seizure activities, a normal EEG will not exclude seizures as a cause of the episodic behavioural or psychiatric symptoms.

Clinicians faced with a patient with post-encephalitis episodic neuro-psychiatric or behavioural symptoms such as aggression, sexual disinhibition or severe emotional lability usually consider seizures and HSE behavioural complications as the main differential diagnoses. Associated symptoms such as urinary incontinence, short-duration self-limiting attacks or a positive EEG will strongly suggest an epileptic focus.

Fortunately, antiepileptic medications are the first line of management for both conditions. Carbamazepine is not only a first-line antiepileptic drug but it is also recognised to possess potent antipsychotic properties. Patients usually respond to relatively small doses of antiepileptic medications and it is unusual that maximum doses or combined therapy will be required. Some of these patients will already be on other medications such as antipsychotic drugs or antidepressants to try to control their symptoms. Discontinuation of these medications may be needed, not only because they can reduce the seizure threshold but also because of their effect on other cognitive function. Antipsychotic drugs in particular cause significant deterioration of confusion, with subsequent worsening of aggression.

If seizure activity is the main pathology, response to antiepileptic drugs is dramatic. In some patients, the picture might be muddled by a background of confusion and disorientation. Clinicians may find it difficult to evaluate their patient's responses to antiepileptic drugs, and a chart of antecedent, behaviour and consequences (ABC) before and after initiation of the therapy will be very valuable as they will provide an objective assessment tool to measure the patient's response to the medication.

The diagnosis of epilepsy will have a substantial impact on the patient's life, especially with issues such as driving or employment. The duration of antiepileptic therapy will also depend on whether it is epilepsy or psychiatric complications of HSE. Therefore, it is important to establish the diagnosis in the most objective way possible. In most cases, diagnosis based on clinical judgement is sufficient. A referral to a specialist epilepsy unit for full assessment will be required in selected cases to confirm or refute the diagnosis.

Further reading:

Hokanen, L., Launes, J. (1997). Cognitive recovery instead of decline after acute encephalitis: a prospective follow up study. *J Neurol Neurosurg Psychiatry* **63**, 222–227.

Kennedy, P. G. E., Chaudhuri, A. (2002). Herpes simplex encephalitis. *J Neurol Neurosurg Psychiatry* **73**, 237–238.

Vallini, A. D., Burns, R. L. (1987). Carbamezepine as therapy for psychiatric sequel of herpes simplex encephalitis. *South Med J* **80**, 1590–1592.

Hypopituitarism following brain injury

A 22-year-old man recovered well from a severe traumatic head injury. During a follow-up appointment eight months after the onset, he complained of the classic cognitive complications of head injury; short-term memory loss, attention and high executive function impairments and minor behavioural problems. The patient mentioned his lack of sex drive and inability to have penile erections. Hypopituitarism was suspected.

Comments

In the acute stage following head injury, elevation or reduction of the pituitary hormonal levels is often a normal physiological response to the severe trauma. A classic hormonal response will show an elevation of the adrenocorticotrophic hormone (ACTH), prolactin and growth hormone (GH) and normal or reduced levels of thyroid-stimulating hormone (TSH), luteinising hormone (LH) and follicle-stimulating hormone (FSH). Patients with very severe head injuries may have reduced levels of ACTH, GH and prolactin and these hormonal deficiencies may contribute to the very poor outcome and high mortality in such patients. Postmortem examinations in these patients have revealed a high incidence of hypothalamic–pituitary damage and have subsequently raised the awareness of pituitary hormonal dysfunction as an important correctable clinical complication of injury. The normal hormonal response to injury usually settles following the acute stage but the time frame for the pituitary function to normalise is unknown and it can range from days to months.

The risk of developing long-term hypopituitarism seems to depend mainly on the severity of the head injury. It is very difficult to extrapolate accurate epidemiological data from the literature as the case mix in the relevant studies does not allow for any conclusive figures to guide clinical practice. A commonsense approach to tackle this problem would be to screen all patients with significantly severe head injuries, especially patients with persistent symptoms that are consistent with deficiency of one or more of the pituitary hormones.

Panhypopituitarism is uncommon following head injury. Deficiencies of FSH/LH, TSH, ACTH or GH are the most common and are also the most significant hormonal deficiencies from a clinical standpoint. Antidiuretic hormone deficiency following head injury is surprisingly rare with the literature suggesting an incidence of less than 1% following severe head injury. Diagnosis of deficiency of antidiuretic hormone is relatively easy as the clinical picture and biochemical abnormalities are unique and the patient response to intranasal desmopressin is usually dramatic.

It is difficult to imagine a head injury complication that is as easy as hypopituitarism to correct. So, why is it unusual for a brain injury rehabilitation service to have clear protocols to guide screening for hypopituitarism?

Endocrinologists insist that for hypopituitarism to be diagnosed, *dynamic tests* should always be performed. The combined pituitary stimulation test is the standard method to evaluate suspected pituitary dysfunction. The patient's pituitary hormones are stimulated using insulin-induced hypoglycaemia. Failure of the pituitary hormones to respond to that stress is diagnostic of hypopituitarism. The test is potentially dangerous and life threatening. It is contraindicated in patients with heart conditions or epilepsy. Considering these facts, it is easy to understand the reluctance of the rehabilitation clinicians to request this test, especially as many patients with head injuries will be susceptible to seizures or further hypoglycaemia-induced brain damage. Acquiring consent from such patients for the test could also be a contentious issue, as many patients with cognitive or communication problems may find it difficult to weight the potential benefits and risks of the test.

Many clinicians are taking a more pragmatic approach to evaluate the head injury patient suspected of having hypopituitarism. Table 3.1 summarises the approach suggested by Bondanelli *et al.* (2005) in their review of the issue. The authors considered all the literature available and felt that a history of severe head injury in conjunction with a clinical picture consistent with pituitary hormonal deficiency should allow the diagnosis to be made if unequivocal results from the standard hormonal essays were found. A special case can be made for GH as its deficiency leads to a clinical presentation that is almost identical to the classic physical and cognitive sequelae of brain injury. Low levels of GH always need to be assessed with a stimulation test. Some authors feel that GH-releasing hormone plus arginine stimulation test could be used instead of the unacceptably dangerous insulin stimulation test. If dynamic tests were needed, several precautions should be implemented to ensure accurate results (Table 3.2).

Table 3.1. Evaluation of key pituitary hormones following head injury

Hormonal deficiency	Clinical presentation	Basic hormonal test	Dynamic tests	Need for hormonal replacement
Growth hormone	Indistinguishable from common features of brain injury in adults, with symptoms such as fatigue and poor attention; impaired growth in children	Single high growth hormone measurement excludes deficiency	Essential to make the diagnosis in most cases; insulin tolerance test is the gold standard; growth hormone-releasing hormone and arginine test may be an alternative	Always needed before puberty; not needed in acute stage following injury; replacement in adults and monitoring effects
Gonadotrophin	Sexual dysfunction in adult patients (e.g. impotence in males and amenorrhoea in females)	Low morning testosterone (oestradiol in females) levels in the absence of raised luteinising hormone (Follicle-stimulating hormone in females) are diagnostic	Not needed	Hormonal replacement not usually needed in the post-acute stage but strongly recommended in chronic deficiency
Thyroid-stimulating hormone	Classic features of hypothyroidism (e.g tiredness, cold intolerence)	Low thyroxine in the absence of raised thyroid-stimulating hormone is diagnostic	Not needed	Hormonal replacement is mandatory in the post-acute and chronic phases
Adrenocortico-trophic hormone	Classic features of adrenal insufficiency (e.g hypotension, hypoglycaemia, electrolyte imbalance)	Morning cortisol: low is diagnostic; low–normal requires dynamic tests	Needed if cortisol level is low–normal: the adrenocorticotrophic hormone test	Hormonal replacement is mandatory in the post-acute and chronic phases

Table 3.2. Requirements for a valid pituitary function assessment

Always consult laboratory before taking samples
Time of sampling should be written on the request form
Some drugs may interfere with the results especially cortisol levels
For dynamic tests:
- insert a large cannula and infuse saline to keep the vein open
- do not use heparin as it may interfere with some hormonal essays
- Wait for 30 minutes before taking the first sample to eliminate the stress of venepuncture as a cause of high hormonal levels
- For each sample, disconnect saline, withdraw and discard 2 ml of the saline and blood mixture then take the sample reconnect saline

Insulin tolerance test can be extremely dangerous; only do if essential

If hormonal deficiencies were diagnosed, hormonal replacement should be considered for all patients. Occasionally, the hormonal deficiency resolves spontaneously after a period of months or years. Therefore, a review of the patient and reevaluation of the diagnosis should be planned for at least the following few years. Patient's response to GH replacement in particular should be evaluated in the most objective way, as some patients will not benefit from GH replacement therapy and the need to continue the hormonal replacement therapy should be revisited.

Reference

Bondanelli, M., Ambrosi, M. R., Zatelli, M. C., *et al.* (2005). Hypopituitarism after traumatic brain injury. *Eur J Endocrinol* **152**, 679–691.

Further reading

Chigo, E., Masel, B., Aimaretti, G., *et al.* (2005). Consensus guidelines on screening for hypopituitarism following traumatic brain injury. *Brain Injury* **19**, 711–724.

Anxiety following head injury

A 28-year-old woman had a traumatic brain injury secondary to a road traffic accident when she was a passenger in a head-on collision. She lost consciousness for a few minutes. However, the post-traumatic amnesia period was four days. She did not have fits following the accident and the CT scan showed no abnormality.

At six weeks after the accident, the patient had a multitude of symptoms and problems. She complained of very poor short-term memory and short attention span. She also found it very difficult to concentrate on tasks like housework. There were a few physical symptoms, such as occasional headaches, dizziness and visual disturbance. The patient described this visual disturbance as a strange feeling that the light was too bright and that the objects she was looking at seemed strange and with odd shapes. The patient also had some problems with coordination in her body and felt woozy or drunk occasionally. She described her gait as unsteady and as if she has 'jelly legs' or that she is walking on a mattress. She said her upper limbs are also affected with feeling that 'they are not fitting properly to my body'. Neurological examination was entirely normal.

The patient was concerned that the head injury was very severe and was leading to complex physical and cognitive problems that would make returning to work very difficult. She was asking for explanations and prognosis.

Comment

Mental health problems are common following head injury. Depression is a high-profile problem that has attracted significant interest from clinicians. It can affect 15 to 45% of patients following traumatic brain injury and is usually associated with poorer outcomes. A major difficulty is the overlap between the cognitive symptoms of depression and the common sequelae of brain injury such as post-concussion syndrome. The main somatic symptom of depression is pain, which usually present with headaches, low-back pain or non-specific generalised aches.

Anxiety can also affect a significant number of patients following brain injury. Literature suggests an incidence of 10–20% for anxiety disorders following traumatic head injury. Post-traumatic stress disorder (PTSD) had been traditionally the anxiety disorder with the strongest association, particularly in that the milder the head injury the more common PTSD becomes. Identifying patients with PTSD is usually straightforward, with patients complaining of flash backs, nightmares about the incident or avoidance of aspects of the incident including places or individuals.

Other common anxiety disorders are panic disorder and general anxiety disorder. The two disorders can present with a combination of cognitive, mood and/or physical symptoms. Patients rarely volunteer information about their mood or panic attacks and they usually concentrate on the physical aspects of the illness, mainly to seek reassurance about the nature and prognosis of the symptoms (Table 3.3).

Table 3.3. Common anxiety disorders

Disorders	Characteristics
Panic disorder	Unexpected and repeated panic attacks with intense anxiety between attacks
General anxiety disorder	Chronic, exaggerated worry and tension that is unfounded or much more severe than the normal anxiety most people experience
Post-traumatic stress disorder	A debilitating anxiety disorder that may develop following a terrifying event; it is characterised by persistent frightening thoughts and memories of the ordeal
Obsessive–compulsive disorder	Recurrent, unwanted thoughts (obsessions) or rituals (compulsions) that feel uncontrollable to the sufferer

There is occasionally a family history of mental health problems (depression and/or anxiety) and patients may give a history of either depression or anxiety before the head injury. They may also admit to having a worrying or obsessive personality in general.

Symptoms are usually bizarre, and pain (which is the usual psychosomatic manifestation of depression) is uncommon. Depersonalisation and derealisation are common presentations. As symptoms of anxiety usually overlap with symptoms secondary to head injury, patients usually use descriptions such as weakness or imbalance to describe depersonalisation or complain of visual problems or photophobia to describe derealisation. Clinicians should encourage patients to elaborate more on these symptoms and offer alternative ways to describe them. They should also enquire about symptoms of panic such as sweating, palpitations or shortness of breath. Patients with general anxiety disorder can present with similar but more persistent symptoms (Table 3.4).

It is important to recognise symptoms of anxiety disorders as they are relatively easy to manage and successful management usually improves cognitive function.

Explanation of the symptoms is an important first step. Some patients will have a catastrophisation cognition, and strong and continuing reassurance is required. Some patients will need formal cognitive–behavioural therapy especially patients with persistent negative thoughts. Techniques taught to the patients include relaxation techniques and distraction.

Antidepressants are the standard treatment for all anxiety disorders, with citalopram the first selective serotonin reuptake inhibitor (SSRI) licensed in the UK for the treatment of panic attacks.

Patients should be warned that they may experience worsening of the symptoms when starting SSRIs. This worsening of symptoms usually improves in a week or two. Patients should not expect improvement of symptoms for

Table 3.4. Presentations of depersonalisation and derealisation

	Characteristics
Depersonalisation	A frightening and/or disturbing experience of not being within one's own body or of being in immediate danger of vanishing/separating from reality – often described as the sensation of living inside a dream; although cognitive functioning remains intact, the sufferers feel disconnected from their sense of self and often interpret it 'as if I am losing my mind'
Derealisation	A state of consciousness that creates a sense of detachment from all environments, as if a plate of glass is in between the mind and the physical world; any concentration requires tremendous effort, and the harder the sufferer tries to focus, the more disconnected they become; it often including feelings of déjà vu or jamais vu. and familiar places look alien, bizarre, and surreal

two or three weeks after initiation of the medication. They should not start with the full therapeutic dose: *start low and go slow*.

The prognosis for anxiety is generally good, with most patients improving with reassurance. Medications such as SSRIs should be continued for at least 12 months to prevent rebound symptoms.

Further reading

Bowen, A., Neumann, W., Conner, M., *et al.* (1998). Mood disorders following traumatic brain injury: identifying the extent of the problem and the people at risk. *Brain Injury* **12**, 177–190.

Simeone, D., Knutelska, M., Nelson, D. (2003). Feeling unreal: a depersonalisation disorder update of 117 cases. *J Clin Psychiatry* **64**, 990–997.

Hydrocephalus following subarachnoid haemorrhage

A 55-year-old woman presented with subarachnoid haemorrhage (SAH) caused by bleeding from an aneurysm of the anterior communicating artery. The aneurysm was clipped surgically and the patient had an uneventful postoperative period. The patient was transferred to the rehabilitation unit 10 days following the onset.

The patient was immobile and doubly incontinent. She was disorientated and seemed very slow in her reactions. A CT scan showed enlarged ventricles.

Comments

More than 80% of SAH follows saccular aneurysms. These aneurysms are not congenital but they develop throughout life, with hypertension, smoking and excessive alcohol intake being the main precipitating factors for their development and rupture. Approximately 4% of the population has significant intracerebral saccular aneurysms and their size, location and shape can provide an indication of the risk of their rupture in the future so surgical ablation could be considered accordingly. Saccular aneurysms are usually located in the base of the brain and affect particular locations within the circle of Lewis. Saccular aneurysms are occasionally associated with cerebral arteriovenous malformations. Such aneurysms are usually located away from the base of the brain within the cerebrum. Their rupture usually results in intracerebral bleeding instead of SAH. The aneurysms result from the increasing arterial flow secondary to the arteriovenous malformation, which weakens the proximal arterial wall. Of patients with an SAH, 10% will not have an identifiable origin (non-aneurysmal perimesencephalic SAH) and the prognosis in this group is usually good. Other rare causes of SAH include cervical arteriovenous malformations, mycotic aneurysms, myxomas, arterial dissection, cocaine abuse and trauma.

Patients presenting with SAH caused by aneurysmal rupture should have their ruptured aneurysm secured, as almost a third of the patients are at risk of rebleeding seven to ten days following the initial bleed. The aneurysm is usually managed surgically or endovascularly. Clipping the aneurysm is the standard surgical management; however, endovascular coiling is gaining popularity and the choice of procedure usually depends on the location of the aneurysm, the condition of the patient and the surgical skills and facilities available.

Acute global ischaemia, acute hydrocephalus and rebleeding are the main fatal complications in the acute stage. Of these, acute global ischaemia is the most common cause of death. Acute hydrocephalus and rebleeding could be successfully managed neurosurgically in selected patients.

Hydrocephalus and secondary cerebral ischaemia are the most common post-acute complications. Secondary cerebral ischaemia usually occurs in the first or second week after aneurysmal SAH in up to one third of patients. Ensuring adequate fluid intake and avoidance of antihypertensive drugs can help in the prevention of secondary ischaemia. Calcium channel antagonists, especially nimodipine, have been shown to reduce the incidence of secondary ischaemia following SAH.

Most patients will have evidence of hydrocephalus in the acute stage, as the presence of blood in the subarachnoid space causes inflammatory arachnoiditis and subsequent slowness of CSF absorption from the arachnoid villi. As the patients are usually very unwell at that stage, the classic picture of normal pressure hydrocephalus (NPH), with the triad of dementia, incontinence and gait apraxia, is rarely seen. Most patients in the post-acute stage following SAH are still immobile and incontinent. The best clinical indication of the presence of significant NPH is the slowness of responses and the general condition of the patient from a cognitive and behavioural standpoint. The patients are sleepy most of the time and despite being able to provide occasional appropriate answers to straightforward questions, they are very slow. A CT scan of the head usually shows enlargement of the ventricles, with occasional enlargement of the temporal horns and sulcal obliteration.

Many patients will have a clinical picture and radiological findings consistent with NPH following SAH or brain injury in general, especially secondary to trauma. The main challenge is to select the patients who are most likely to respond to shunt insertion. Several tests, such as the tap test, intracranial pressure monitoring, CSF infusion tests and external lumbar CSF drainage, are available to support the decision-making process. Unfortunately, these tests have low sensitivity and are unable to provide conclusive evidence to predict the success of a shunt insertion.

In the tap test, the clinical picture and cognitive abilities are monitored before withdrawal of 40–50 ml of CSF. The changes in the patient's cognitive abilities as measured by objective cognitive function tests and as observed subjectively by the staff dealing with the patient are documented. A significant improvement would predict favourable outcome of shunt insertion. The value of the test in patients with an SAH or brain injury is not well established. Many patients have considerable cognitive impairment secondary to their brain injury, which will mask any significant change following the tap test. The low sensitivity of the test was demonstrated in a study where it was used with patients with idiopathic NPH (Marmarou *et al.*, 2005).

Patients with NPH frequently have normal intracranial pressure. However, monitoring over a 24-hour period may reveal significant abnormalities, that could indicate poor cerebral compliance.

The main objective of the CSF infusion test is to determine the arachnoid villi resistance to CSF absorption. Lumbar puncture needles are inserted in two sites, with normal saline infused from one needle and the rate of increase of the CSF pressure recorded from the other.

Assessment of external lumbar CSF drainage is probably the most sensitive and specific method to predict the response to shunting. In this test, a controlled removal of CSF is maintained throughout 24 hours and the clinical response monitored.

A tap test can be done in some rehabilitation settings. From my experience, in severely affected patients after SAH or brain injury, the changes following CSF withdrawal are modest in most of the patients, and many of these will go on to respond very well to shunt insertion. Other tests such as CSF infusion tests are usually carried out in the neurosurgery department, giving the neurosurgeons a better chance to assemble the various evidence, with the final clinical decision guided by the results of the clinical, radiological, intracranial pressure and infusion tests.

Ventriculo-peritoneal shunts are the standard system used in most centres to manage hydrocephalus. Early complications of the procedure include bleeding, infection, shunt obstruction and over or under drainage of CSF. In the rehabilitation period, shunt malfunction is usually caused by infection or hardware failure, with the valve or proximal or distal catheter malfunctioning. Acute shunt dysfunction usually presents with a dramatic picture: the patient complaining of severe headache, photophobia and vomiting, with rapid deterioration of consciousness level. Urgent revision of the shunt is essential.

The clinical presentation of a patient with a partially obstructed shunt is less dramatic. Headaches and deterioration of cognitive function and mobility are common complaints. An infected shunt must be revised as it is extremely difficult to eradicate a colonised bacterial or fungal shunt infection.

Reference

Marmarou, A., Bergsneider, M., Klinge, P., et al. (2005). The value of supplemental prognostic tests for the preoperative assessment of idiopathic normal pressure hydrocephalus. *Neurosurgery* **57** (Suppl. 2), 17–28.

Further reading

Czosnyke, M., Whitfield, P. (2006). Hydrocephalus. A practical guide to CSF dynamics and ventriculoperitoneal shunts. *Adv Clin Neurosci Rehabil* **6**,14–17.

Van Gijn, J., Rinkel, G. J. (2001). Subarachnoid haemorrhage: diagnosis, causes and management. *Brain* **124**, 249–278.

Autonomic impairment following brain injury

A 22-year-old man had a severe head injury following a motorcycle accident. A brain CT scan showed minor changes and diffuse axonal injury was suggested. Three weeks later, the patient remained in a low consciousness state and was managed conservatively in the intensive care unit, where he had episodes of hyperpyrexia, tachycardia, tachypnoea and hypertension. During these episodes, the patient assumed an extensor posturing. The duration of these episodes ranged from a few minutes to more than 12 hours. Comprehensive tests excluded sepsis, cardiac abnormalities and pulmonary embolism as the causes of these episodes.

Comments

Autonomic dysreflexia is a well-recognised complication of high spinal cord injury. In this condition, patients present with a sudden sympathetic storm, with severe hypertension, tachycardia and tachypnoea. An irritant such as an obstructed urinary catheter or a painful stimulus often precipitates the attacks. Autonomic dysreflexia is a life-threatening condition and prompt medical management is needed to control the high blood pressure and prevent serious complications such as pulmonary oedema or stroke.

Patients with severe head injury can present with a similar picture. Unfortunately, the literature presents only few case reports or small case series. There is no consensus what this syndrome should be called. Names such as dysautonomia, autonomic dysfunction syndrome, autonomic storming or paroxysmal autonomic instability with dystonia have been used. The syndrome is more common in patients with hypoxic or diffuse axonal brain damage and it is more common in patients with prolonged periods of low consciousness state.

Direct damage to the temperature, respiratory and blood pressure regulating centres in the thalamus or hypothalamus is unusual. It is believed that the cortical, subcortical or brainstem autonomic controlling centres are the usual sites where the primary damage takes place, with subsequent release phenomenon in the thalamic and hypothalamic major autonomic centres leading to temperature, respiratory and blood pressure dysregulation. The muscle rigidity, dystonia or extensor posturing are probably caused by a different mechanism affecting mainly the brainstem inhibitory signals to the spinal cord, resulting in a hyperexcitable spinal cord reflexes.

The complexity of the post brain injury dysautonomia syndrome is reflected by the variety of pharmacological agents that have been used to control it. The rational of using beta blockers such as propranolol or alpha blockers such as clonidine is obvious. Blockade of either alpha- or beta-adrenoceptors (or both) should counteract the excessive sympathetic stimulation leading to symptoms such as tachycardia and hypertension. Both dopamine agonists such as bromocriptine and different dopamine antagonists have been used in attempts to control the muscular symptoms such as rigidity and dystonia. The results have been disappointing with both groups.

The use of such contradictory methods to control the same group of symptoms indicates the lack of a coherent approach in the management of the syndrome in the available literature.

Morphine sulphate action on central opioid receptors leads to bradycardia, hypotension and depression of respiratory rate. This unique action makes the morphine derivatives the most commonly used drugs to control the symptoms of dysautonomia. In general, it is clear from the literature that the treating physicians use a pragmatic approach in the management of the symptoms, using a particular drug to control a specific problem or group of symptoms, for example using beta blockers to control tachycardia and paracetamol to control fever. Similar to autonomic dysreflexia in spinal cord injury, dysautonomia following brain injury can be fatal. Manifestations of the syndrome should be aggressively managed, preferably in an intensive care setting.

The literature clearly shows that brain-injured patients presenting with paroxysmal dysautonomia have poor prognosis. This is not surprising as the syndrome affects patients with severe brain injury and no attempts have been made to compare the affected patients with another group of brain-injured patients with similar pathology and severity of brain injury. It is rare to see paroxysmal dysautonomia in the chronic phase of brain injury even if the consciousness state remained low.

As post brain injury dysautonomia has several differential diagnoses, it is difficult to estimate the real incidence of the syndrome. Sepsis, neuroleptic malignant syndrome, diencephalic seizures, central fever and other medical and surgical causes such as bone fractures should all be excluded. Blackman *et al.* (2004) have suggested specific criteria for the diagnosis of the dysautonomia syndrome (Table 3.5). The most important criterion is probably

Table 3.5. Criteria for diagnosis of paroxysmal autonomic instability with dystonia after brain injury as suggested by Blackman *et al.* (2004)

Criteria[a]
Severe head injury
Fever $> 38.5°C$
Pulse $> 130/min$
Respiratory rate $> 40/min$
Agitation
Diaphoresis
Dystonia

[a] The duration is at least one cycle a day for at least three days. Other conditions must be excluded.

exclusion of all possible treatable causes of fever, tachycardia and tachypnoea with dystonia and rigidity. The criteria were suggested after examination of a small number of their patients (seven) and the cases reported in the literature (incomplete data of 71 cases).

Reference

Blackman, J. A., Patrick, P. D., Buck, M. L., Rust, J. R. (2004). Paroxysmal autonomic instability with dystonia after brain injury. *Arch Neurol* **61**, 321–328.

Further reading

Baguley, I. J., Nicols, J. N., Felmingham, K. L., *et al.* (1999). Dysautonomia after traumatic brain injury: A forgotten syndrome. *J Neurol Neurosurg Psychiatry* **67**, 39–43.

Locked-in syndrome

A 32-year-old woman presented with a sudden onset of severe headache and confusion, which progressed quickly to a profound impaired consciousness level. When presenting to the medical admission unit, her Glasgow Coma Score was 3/15; she assumed a decerebrate posture and had an apnoeic episode. The patient was intubated and artificially ventilated. An MRI scan suggested the diagnosis of a basilar artery thrombosis. The diagnosis was confirmed with MRI angiography. Diagnosis of a locked-in syndrome was suspected because of the anatomical location of the lesion. Attempts to communicate with the patient using eye movements gave unreliable yes/no responses initially. However, a few weeks later the responses became more consistent and a rehabilitation programme was commenced.

Comments

Many working parties have tried to suggest clear-cut definitions to help clinicians to differentiate with confidence between coma, vegetative state and locked-in syndrome (Andrews, 1999) (Table 3.6). Such efforts are extremely valuable in the clinical setting as prognosis and management of these conditions differ substantially. Accurate differentiation should also support decision making relevant to the complex ethical and medicolegal issues that are commonly present with such cases.

Diagnosis of these conditions is rarely absolutely certain, and most patients will need careful and prolonged periods of assessment to clarify the diagnosis.

Table 3.6. Differentiation of consciousness states[a]

State	Characteristics
Coma	A state of unconsciousness in which the patient shows no or minimal response to stimuli, has no sleep/awake pattern and no eye opening; brainstem reflexes are maintained
Vegetative state	Low consciousness state in which the patient maintains sleep/awake cycles, can have spontaneous eye opening and may respond to pain; there is no awareness of the surrounding environment and no ablity to interact with it in any meaningful manner; persistent vegetative state can be used to describe patients who have been in a vegetative state for more than 30 days

[a] Diagnoses of brain death, coma, vegetative state and locked-in syndrome are made on clinical grounds. Tests such as electroencephalography can play an important role to support the diagnosis.

In many cases, there might be an overlap between two conditions or the patient will fluctuate between the features of different conditions.

Locked-in syndrome is usually caused by a vascular or a traumatic event. Basilar artery occlusion is the most common cause but pontine haemorrhage is also common. Locked-in syndrome caused by trauma is often associated with cognitive impairment, which can complicate the process of assessment or rehabilitation. Demyelination, infections and tumours are rare causes of the syndrome.

Some authors classify locked-in syndrome as *classic, incomplete or total*. In the classic syndrome, the patient suffers from tertraplegia and anarthria with preserved consciousness and vertical eye movements. In the incomplete syndrome, the patient will have some added voluntary movements other than eye movements, which may make a huge difference to the patients potential for rehabilitation. The total locked-in syndrome is the most catastrophic as the patient will have no way to communicate despite having normal consciousness.

This classification demonstrates the difficulty in establishing communication with some patients either because of their cognitive impairment or because of the inability to generate voluntary eye movement. Consequently, it is not unusual for some patients to be diagnosed as having a vegetative state for months or years and in further assessment found to have locked-in syndrome.

Once the diagnosis of locked-in syndrome is made, a reliable way to communicate with the patient should be established. A yes/no response from the patient is usually communicated via eye movement. Patients with incomplete locked-in syndrome may be able to use other body movements to communicate. Many patients will struggle to achieve reliable and consistent

Table 3.7. Requirements for accurate assessment of consciousness state and communication

Exclude relevant pathologies such as severe cognitive impairment
Ensure medical stability including adequate rehydration and nutrition
Involve family and all staff in the assessment process; any sign of voluntary action should be documented and discussed with the rest of the team; the family are often the first to notice significant signs
Consider fluctuations as a cause for inconsistency of abilities
Review posture to facilitate the patient's ability to mobilise specific muscles intentionally
Reduce sensory stimulation especially when trying to assess the patient
Review medications especially sedating agents

responses especially in the early stages after the onset. This should not discourage the rehabilitation team from continuing to work with the patient to try to improve the reliability and accuracy of the responses. Communicating with the patient will provide an excellent opportunity to assess the patient's psychological state and to provide support to help in coping with such devastating disability (Table 3.7).

Many methods to improve communication further should be tried. Communication aids could be incorporated within an environmental control system. However, a simple aid should be tried first and then other commands and controls added in due course as the patient becomes more skilled in using the aid.

Bioengineers and clinicians are now collaborating in the development of a new exciting technology that might facilitate better communication with patients with locked-in syndrome. Computer–brain interface refers to a direct pathway between the human brain and an external device. The signals from the brain can be picked up by either an invasive or a non-invasive method. Most of the research so far has used invasive methods; however, most practical applications use a non-invasive method based mainly on EEG signals. The main problem impeding such promising technology is its complexities and the difficulties the patients face in learning to operate such systems. Therefore, most of the research so far has concentrated on patients with high spinal injuries as such patients are easy to communicate with and teach, especially with such complex technology.

Reference

Andrews, K. (1999). The vegetative state: clinical diagnosis. *Postgrad Med J* **75**, 321–324.

Further reading

Smith, E., Delargy, M. (2005). Locked in syndrome *BMJ* **330**, 406–409.

Dobkin, B. H. (2007). Brain–computer interface technology as a tool to augment plasticity and outcomes for neurological rehabilitation. *J Physiol* **579**, 637–642.

Pharmacological management of attention impairment

A 23-year-old man had a severe head injury that left him with complex physical and cognitive problems. After six months, the patient's attentional deficits had a major impact on the management of his other disabilities. The patient had a very low level of arousal and his attention span was very short. Attention impairments affected the reliability of communication and memory and the patient's ability to participate in therapy sessions.

Comments

Impairments of attention, memory and higher executive function are the classic triad of the non-localising cognitive sequelae following any type of brain injury. Attention deficits are probably the most important of the three, as poor attention will impact on almost all cognitive and functional tasks performed by the patient. Many clinicians believe that post-traumatic amnesia is a confusional state resulting mainly from attention impairment. The patient's poor attention leads to his inability to retain information during a period, with subsequent failure to remember events from that period. Many long-term cognitive impairments such as impulsivity and rigidity of thoughts are predominantly caused by attentional deficits.

Attention is regarded as a multifaceted concept that is controlled by a network of diverse brain structures. Several centres in the prefrontal area, the thalamus and the brainstem are linked by the reticular activating system and are believed to play a major role in maintaining attention. There is also evidence of asymmetry between the two hemispheres, with the non-dominant hemisphere playing a more prominent role in attention function.

Backward digit span and seven subtraction tests are commonly used by physicians to screen for attention deficits. Formal psychological tests can assess the different components of attention function. The main components of attention are *arousal, focused attention, divided attention* and *speed of information processing*. Accurate estimation of each component is not essential in the clinical setting as they poorly reflect the difficulties the patient faces in everyday tasks.

Three different strategies to improve attention could be integrated in a standard brain injury rehabilitation programme: attention-retraining programmes, extensive practice of functional tasks and pharmacological interventions.

There is sufficient evidence to recommend attention-retraining programmes especially in the post-acute phase. During the acute phase following brain injury, there is insufficient evidence available to distinguish between the genuine beneficial effects of such programmes and the natural recovery during that phase. Most attention-training programmes are now computer based and relatively easy to administer.

Extensive practice of functional tasks is extremely difficult to evaluate using robust research methodology. However, the consensus of experts and many non-randomised trials support its routine use.

Methylphenidate is the drug most commonly used in patients with attention problems following brain injury. As an amphetamine, it was first used by pilots during World War Two to improve concentration and vigilance. Later, it was used extensively to treat depression. The arrival of the tricyclic antidepressants in the late 1960s marked the end of the golden era of amphetamines in general. At present, methylphenidate is used mainly for narcolepsy and attention-deficit hyperactive disorder in children. It is that last indication that brought methylphenidate to the attention of clinicians working with brain-injured patients as children with attention-deficit hyperactive disorder and brain-injured patients with attention deficits have many similarities. The safety of methylphenidate has also been studied extensively because of its use in children. Most paediatricians feel that the notoriety of methylphenidate is unjustified as most symptoms commonly attributed to the drug are actually preexisting characteristics of the affected children and improve with stimulant treatment. Another myth related to methylphenidate is its potential to cause seizures. Several studies have shown that the drug can be safely used in brain-injured patients, even those at high risk of seizures, as it is associated with a trend toward reduction rather than increase in seizure frequency.

Many studies have shown methylphenidate to be effective in brain-injured adults with attention deficits. Unfortunately, most studies were not controlled and many had serious methodological flaws. All the studies tested the use of methylphenidate for a very short period of time and no data are available regarding the efficacy or safety of its long-term use. There is a general agreement, however, that methylphenidate mainly improves speed of information processing and arousal. On a functional level, a few reports have suggested beneficial effects of methylphenidate on behaviour, with reduction in the frequency and severity of anger outbursts and impulsiveness.

The interest in methylphenidate as a useful agent in brain injury did not only focus on its well-proven stimulant role it was also proposed that it may possess a *neuroprotective* action. Neurochemical events following brain injury include an acute excitotoxic phase and a post-acute phase characterised by neuronal hypofunction. It has been suggested that neurostimulants enhance functional recovery during that second phase, by preventing or reversing an injury-induced remote functional depression of catecholamine levels and turnover in the brain tissue and/or alleviating metabolic remote functional depression by increasing responsivity of the remaining neuronal pathways.

A few studies have tried to test this assumption using different amphetamines (methylphenidate or dexedrine) for a few weeks following traumatic brain injury or stroke – to coincide with the presumed narrow window of opportunity in the post-acute stage. Most of these studies had poor methodologies and their results were mixed and it is impossible to interpret their results. Any improvement can be explained by either the normal recovery process or by methylphenidate enhancement of attention and mood, with a subsequent facilitation of the patient's participation with the rehabilitation programme.

Other neurostimulants such as amantadine and bromocriptine have been used, particularly for patients suffering from unilateral visual spatial neglect, but the results are not conclusive. Modafinil is a eugenic drug (which mainly means 'good arousal'). Its mode of action is not well understood. It seems that it has a central adrenergic effect at α_1-adrenoceptors and also an antagonist action at GABA (gamma-aminobutyric acid) receptors. Modafinil is licensed for narcolepsy and almost any disorder causing sleepiness or somnolence. There is anecdotal evidence that this drug can lead to improvement in a selected group of brain-injured patients who mainly have problems with arousal.

Further reading

Glenn, M. B. (1998). Methylphenidate for cognitive and behavioural dysfunction after traumatic brain injury. *J Head Trauma Rehabil* **5**, 87–90.

Plenger, P. M., Dixon, C. E., Castillo, R. M., et al. (1996). Subacute methyl-phenidate treatment for moderate to severe traumatic brain injury: a preliminary double blind placebo controlled study. *Arch Phys Med Rehabil* **77**, 536–540.

Whyte, J., Rose, T., Glenn, M. B., et al. (1994). Quantification of attention related behaviors in individuals with traumatic brain injury. *Am J Phys Med Rehabil* **73**, 2–9.

Rehabilitation of pontine myelinolysis

A 48-year-old woman with a long-standing drinking problem presented to A&E with a single seizure following two days of progressive confusion. The patient's sodium level was 112 mmol/l on admission. Normal saline was administered to correct this and the following day the patient's sodium level was 129 mmol/l. This correction of the electrolyte imbalance coincided with an improvement in the patient's clinical condition.

Two days later, the patient had a sudden physical and cognitive deterioration with flaccid paralysis affecting the four limbs and reduced consciousness level. A diagnosis of pontine myelinolysis (PM) was suggested.

Comments

Pontine myelinolysis is a rare neurological disorder that predominantly affects the pons but can also affect other areas in the brain such as the thalamus, basal ganglia or cerebellum. Patients with such diffuse demyelination are usually referred to as having **extrapontine myelinolysis**. In PM, the demyelination process is not inflammatory and is mainly a result of a sudden and drastic change in sodium serum levels. In clinical practice, most patients presenting with PM are alcoholics and/or malnourished. It is not clear if this state of chronic ill health predispose patients to PM. Patients with eating disorders or liver transplantations are also vulnerable to PM.

The classic presentation of PM is of a patient with an alcohol problem and seizures or confusion that can be linked to severe hyponatraemia. This is usually treated by saline infusion, which rapidly corrects the serum sodium concentration. The patient's clinical condition improves, but two or three days later they present with dramatic deterioration, with psychiatric symptoms and neurological signs. Quadriparesis and pseudobulbar palsy secondary to corticobulbar and corticospinal tract damage are the impairments most usually seen. However, dystonia, ataxia and other movement disorders have also been reported. Sensory changes are rare. The patient with severe pontine demyelination can present with a locked-in syndrome caused by complete disruption of all the motor tracts running through the pons.

The pathology of PM is not fully understood. Neuroscientists have always been intrigued by PM because of its almost exclusive attack on the pons. One theory proposed that dense mixing of pontine grey and white matter increases the vulnerability of the myelin sheath to toxic attacks. Structures such as the thalamus, which occasionally share the same pathology, have similar histological structure.

Adams first described PM in 1959, and for the following two decades, it was a postmortem diagnosis. That gave the impression that the general outcome of PM is grave. With the arrival of more sophisticated scanning techniques, the diagnosis of PM could be accurately made in the acute stage. There are no comprehensive data on the disease prognosis but the impression is that the prognosis is not as poor as once thought.

The only data available on the outcome of PM come from a study by Menger and Jorge (1999), who examined the outcome of 34 patients with PM, 32 of whom survived. Of these, 11 completely recovered, 11 had some deficits but were independent, and 10 were dependent (four because of disorders of memory or cognition, three with tetraparesis, two with cerebellar ataxia and one with polyneuropathy). The clinical improvement did not correlate with the severity of the disease as measured by MRI.

This study suggests a neurological condition with generally a good prognosis and little worse than other acute demyelinating disorders such as Guillain–Barré syndrome. Even the patients who were left dependent following PM suffered from impairments such as peripheral neuropathy, ataxia or cognitive impairments that could also be attributed to their alcohol dependency.

This general impression about the prognosis is certainly in line with my experience of the rehabilitation of a handful of patients with PM. All of them showed almost full neurological recovery. The main reason for long-term dependence was contractures of large joints caused by severe spasticity in the acute stage.

Unfortunately, most of the literature dealing with PM comments on the pathology and acute management, with little emphasis on the rehabilitation issues facing these patients. Considering the relatively good chance for neurological recovery, aggressive management of the risk factors for long-term disability is paramount. Spasticity should be appropriately managed with medications including botulinum toxin followed by splinting or serial casting if needed. Joint contractures could develop within a very short period of time and it might be too late to act once they are well established. Pseudobulbar palsy often leads to dysphagia. A robust method to maintain the patient's nutritional needs should be established early, especially as most patients suffer from alcoholism or nutritional or eating disorders.

Cognitive and psychiatric impairments are not uncommon following PM. Some authors have suggested that this indicates the significant role that the brainstem plays in maintaining higher cognitive function. This is very difficult to verify as most of the patients suffer from significant long-standing alcohol problems that might be the primary cause of such cognitive and behavioural deterioration. Wernicke's encephalopathy is strongly associated with PM and it may result in such severe higher function deficits. Unfortunately, cognitive and behavioural impairments secondary to PM have never been systematically examined. The data provided by Menger and Jorge (1999) indicate that a significant number of patients with poor outcome are dependent because of their cognitive deficits.

Clinicians treating this disorder should recognise the paradox between the physical and cognitive complications of PM. Aggressive rehabilitation aiming at preventing long-term physical disability is important as neurological recovery is expected in many cases. Additionally, cognitive rehabilitation should be started early as patients' cognitive abilities often fail to improve to their premorbid level.

Reference

Menger, H., Jorge, J. (1999). Outcome of central pontine and extrapontine myelinolysis. *J Neurol* **246**, 700–705.

Further reading

Martin, R. J. (2004). Central pontine and extrapontine myelinolysis: the osmotic demyelination syndromes. *J Neurol Neurosurg Psychiatry* **75**, 22–28.
Mochizuki, H., Masaki, T., Miyakawa, T. (2003). Benign type of central pontine myelinolysis in alcoholism: clinical, neuroradiological and electrophysiological findings. *J Neurol* **250**, 1077–1083.

Assessment of frontal lobe function

A 56-year-old man had a traumatic brain injury after a fall. A CT scan showed bilateral frontal lobe contusion. The patient had post-traumatic amnesia for two days. Five days after the onset, the patient made a full physical recovery and his Mini-Mental State Examination (MMSE) was 29/30. However, staff reported some incidents suggesting disinhibition and occasional disorientation. Additionally, the patient's family expressed their concern, feeling that his behaviour and personality had changed significantly.

Comments

Since the mid-1980s, the MMSE has been increasingly used as the standard tool to screen patients for cognitive impairments during their stay in medical or rehabilitation wards. A major criticism of the MMSE is its insensitivity to the cognitive deficits secondary to frontal lobe damage. As many brain-injured patients will have a clinical presentation consistent with a frontal lobe syndrome, concerns about the suitability of the MMSE to screen such patients is understandable.

As most of the frontal cortex is subcortical white matter, its function is strongly related to the subcortical structures especially the basal ganglia and the thalamus. Therefore, direct damage to the frontal lobes caused by injury or atrophy is not the only recognised pathway by which symptoms of frontal

Table 3.8. Common causes of frontal cognitive impairment

Area affected	Causes
Primarily the frontal lobes	Traumatic brain injury, frontotemporal dementia, hypoxic brain injury, tumours
Primarily the basal ganglia	Lewy body dementia, Parkinson's disease (late in the disease), Huntington's disease, progressive supranuclear palsy, Wilson's disease

Table 3.9. Complications of damage to the specific frontal lobe areas

Area	Deficit
Dorsolateral	Cognitive inflexibility (detected by cognitive tests)
Orbitofrontal	Apathy, abulia
Anterior cingulate	Disinhibition

lobe dysfunction can be initiated. Basal ganglia pathologies are probably a more common cause of frontal lobe dysfunction, with disorders such as Parkinson's disease, Huntington's disease, multisystem atrophy and progressive supranuclear palsy presenting with cognitive impairments comparable with those seen in direct frontal lobe damage. Several subtypes of dementia, such as Lewy body dementia, also present with a similar picture. This group of disorders with pathology affecting mainly the basal ganglia and presenting with dementia are called subcortical dementias. This diversity of causes of frontal lobe syndrome has led some authors to call its cognitive manifestations **frontal/subcortical manifestations** (Table 3.8).

The frontal lobes can be classified into three distinct areas, with damage to each area producing a unique clinical picture and a specific cognitive or behavioural manifestation (Table 3.9). For most patients, the pathology, whether traumatic, vascular, atrophic or neoplastic, will affect the three areas but probably with different severity for each one. Damage to the **dorsolateral prefrontal area** usually produces significant well-defined cognitive deficits that are relatively easy to detect with standard frontal lobe function testing. Damage to the **anterior cingulated area** usually produces apathy and abulia, with symptoms occasionally mistaken for depression. The results of damage to the **orbitofrontal area** is probably the most disabling, with disinhibition and social inappropriate behaviour interfering with the patient's social integration.

Table 3.10. Cognitive testing (dorsolateral frontal lobe)

Function	Test
Attention	Digit span (forward and backwards)
Initiation	Verbal fluency (e.g. spontaneous word generation: more than 17 words starting with 's' in 1 min and more than 13 for 'f')
	Planning (e.g. 'What would you do in a fire or on finding a wallet?)
Abstract thinking	Interpretation of a proverb
	Similarities and differences (e.g. between cow and horse)
Response inhibition and set shifting	Trail-making test Motor sequence tests

With such diverse aetiologies and complex clinical presentations, recognition of the signs of frontal lobe involvement is important, particularly in acute situations such as traumatic brain injury. Many psychological tests are available to evaluate frontal lobe function. The Frontal Assessment Battery (FAB) is probably the most popular. Other general cognitive assessment tools try to address the deficiencies of the MMSE by giving more emphasis to the language and the classic frontal function impairments such as initiation, abstraction and thought flexibility. Addenbrooke's Cognitive Examination (ACE) has proven its value as an excellent screening test, especially for dementia.

To screen adequately for cognitive impairment, clinicians can either use one of the more comprehensive tools such as ACE or use the MMSE and add to it a few tests specifically to exclude frontal function impairments. As MMSE is a standard test and most clinicians have extensive experience in using it, adding a few frontal function assessments might be a more practical approach.

Table 3.10 lists the recommended tests to evaluate frontal lobe function, especially in patients with dorsolateral area damage. Naming tests, particularly the Letter Fluency Test, are probably the most sensitive tests for frontal lobe damage. In all naming tests, dominant temporal lobe (semantics) and frontal lobes (initiation) are used to generate normal responses. When asked for category naming ('Try to come up with as many names of animals as possible in one minute'), a patient with intact language function and semantic library in his dominant temporal lobe will be able to come up with a satisfactory list despite having frontal lobe damage. As the names are held in the semantic library under categories, it is easy for the patient to delve into the needed file and access most of the names needs. In assessing letter fluency, the patient is asked to mention as many names as he or she can that start with a particular letter (usually F, A or S). The patient will be unable to rely on his/her semantic library this time as the words are not indexed alphabetically and the patient must use initiation and attention to generate the requested words. Therefore, letter fluency is considered the most sensitive simple test to exclude significant frontal lobe function impairment.

Some aspects of frontal lobe dysfunction such as disinhibition, apathy, impulsivity or rigidity of thinking are very difficult to assess with formal testing. The patient will almost invariably deny such problems because of poor insight. Indirect history, such as asking about problems at work or in the family, can give some indication to the patient's general behaviour. Interviewing a close relative is extremely helpful. Some informal tests such as the Cognitive Estimates Test may prompt incorrect or bizarre responses with questions such as 'How tall is the Tower of London?' 'How fast is a formula 1 car?' The idea of the test is to ask the patient to estimate a value that he/she is not expected to know but should be able to give a rough estimate for based on extrapolation from other known values of similar objects.

Interpretation of proverbs such as 'a bird in the hand is better than two in the bush' and asking the patient to mention the similarities and differences between two subjects such as a cat and a cow are useful tests for abstract thinking.

The patient's behaviour and the way in which the patient answers the questions should be considered as well. A patient with pure attention deficits might spend some time thinking and trying to find the right response to a Backward Digit Test, while a patient with impulsivity will respond promptly without thinking, but giving a similar false response.

Rehabilitation of patients with frontal lobe symptoms usually concentrates on the environment and carers as patients' limited insight into their difficulties act as a huge barrier to participation with therapy. A patient with pure cognitive impairments can usually cope with a rigid routine and can even maintain employment if the work structure is predictable and with minimal face-to-face contact. Patients with behavioural impairments such as disinhibition are the most difficult to manage and many of them need 24-hour care.

Further reading

Bak, T. (2006). Cognitive profile in Parkinson's syndromes. *Adv Clin Neurosci Rehabil* **6**, 12–14.

Kipps, C. M., Hodges, J. R. (2005). Cognitive assessment for clinicians. *J Neurol Neurosurg Psychiatry* **76**, 22–30.

Stewart, J. T. (2006). The frontal/subcortical dementias. *Geriatrics* **61**, 23–27.

An aggressive patient

A 56-year-old man was admitted following a road traffic accident which resulted in a traumatic brain injury. Initial CT scan revealed extensive damage and he required a craniotomy for evacuation of a subdural haematoma and a left frontal lobectomy. On admission to the neuro-rehabilitation unit, he had no physical deficits; however, he had a range of cognitive, behavioural and emotional problems.

After a few days, the patient requested that he be let out of the ward and allowed to go home as he believed that there was nothing wrong with him. Refusal to meet his requests led to verbal and physical aggression (pushing and hitting staff). At this point, the patient was still disorientated and was incapable of retaining new information. He was taking sedative medication for agitation, a problem that had been previously identified on the high dependency unit.

The frequency and intensity of his aggressive behaviour increased over the next three weeks. Ward staff and other patients became anxious when around him, although some staff were able to calm him and escort him off the ward for brief periods. At the multidisciplinary meeting, the team discussed increasing his sedative medication and using the Mental Health Act to control his behaviour and enforce his detainment on the ward.

Comments

Aggressive behaviour is a common consequence of brain injury, particularly after frontal lobe damage. It may take the form of purely verbal aggression or it may be physical. All forms of aggression can cause distress to staff, carers, relatives and other patients, as well as presenting considerable risk.

Aggression may be related to a number of neuropsychological factors including lack of insight and self-monitoring, impulsivity and comprehension and memory problems. However, there are a number of environmental and psychological factors that may also have an impact upon a patient's aggressive behaviour. Prevention of significant behavioural problems may be achieved through training staff in behavioural management.

Behavioural disturbance following acquired brain injury has often been treated through the use of sedative medication. Although this approach may be necessary in addressing immediate risk situations, the potential for side effects of such medication in patients with brain injuries is high. These negative effects may lead to further impairment of cognitive functioning and a slowing of neuronal recovery, thus impeding rehabilitation and community reintegration. Therefore, alternative means of managing aggression must be considered.

Management of an aggressive patient is always a multidisciplinary team responsibility. Certain professions may take a lead role in coordinating the team's approach (e.g. clinical psychology) because of their training in behavioural management. Any intervention should be based on an assessment that has identified the 'function' of the behaviour (i.e. what is the patient attempting to achieve or communicate through behaviour), as this may not always be obvious. An assessment may follow a 'functional analysis' (or 'ABC analysis') approach that attempts to establish the antecedents (i.e. immediate triggers) of behaviour and the consequences (i.e. immediate benefits of the behaviour to the patient). A more detailed assessment may use the principles of applied behaviour analysis in addressing a wider range of factors impinging upon the behaviour of a neurologically impaired patient.

Once the aggressive behaviour has been identified and assessed, a behavioural management plan should be drawn up to introduce environmental and psychosocial strategies as a first-line approach and to develop rehabilitation goals to address specific neuropsychological deficits. This will help to coordinate staff, relatives and carers in their approach to the behavioural problem. Within the plan, the conditions for utilising physical restraint and pharmacological management strategies may be specified as second-line interventions.

Environmental considerations include provision for privacy and a calming room, facilitating pursuit of personal interests, and structuring routines on the ward to ensure as much meaningful activity for the person as possible.

Psychological strategies include developing communication strategies that all staff can use to meet the patient's communication and cognitive abilities, teaching more appropriate social skills and providing structured and regular education regarding the person's condition and the treatment available. Training in 'de-escalation' (a calming technique) may be provided for staff through the clinical psychology staff or other professionals with skills in behaviour management.

Development of a positive feedback or 'reward' programme that enables the patient to relearn acceptable behaviour and restores some self-esteem should be considered. Occasionally, aggressive behaviour is reinforced through unintended positive consequences (e.g. increased time with staff and relatives, 'soft' talking, conceding to demands). Therefore, a programme designed to reduce positive consequences that maintain the behaviour may also be considered in conjunction with a reward programme.

Education of both staff and relatives regarding behavioural problems following a traumatic brain injury is beneficial in reducing anxiety and developing confidence in handling aggression. Regular team meetings and discussions with the family are helpful in identifying changes in behaviour, updating the behavioural management plan, sharing good practice and providing support in stressful situations.

In severe cases of aggression when there is no time to implement environmental and psychological strategies, physical restraint and/or pharmacological management may be necessary. There are ethical, legal and safety implications of these management strategies and so it is necessary to conduct a risk analysis, to ensure documentation is timely and accurate and to inform relatives and carers of the need for such an approach. In complex medical cases where pharmacological intervention is being considered, psychiatric advice should be sought.

Further reading

LaVigna, G. W., Willis, T. J. (1995). Challenging behavior: a model for breaking the barriers to social and community integration. *positive prac* **1**, 8–15.

Sohlberg, M. M., Mateer, C. A. (2001). Managing challenging behaviors. In Sohlberg, M. M., Mateer, C. A. (eds.), *Cognitive Rehabilitation*, pp. 337–369. New York: Guilford Press.

Progressive neurological disorders

4

During an annual, routine medical review for a patient with a progressive neurological condition such as multiple sclerosis or Parkinson's disease, it is not unusual to hear the patient saying 'what I really need doctor is more physiotherapy'. A referral for further physiotherapy is often made.

It is very difficult to propose the perfect model of service for patients with neurological progressive disorders. However, regular reviews can hardly meet the patient's needs. In my view, what the patient needs is an assessment followed by a prompt intervention to address his/her problem. The expertise and interests of a patient's GP vary greatly and some would prefer to delegate responsibility to a more specialist service. The popularity of specialist nurses is self-evident and they often fulfil their role as a first contact efficiently. They should be able to channel the patient to the appropriate service whether it is for therapy assessment or for medical, nutritional or social review.

One of the shortcomings of this model is the relative lack of experience of the specialist nurses regarding the different roles of all the professionals that can potentially help the patient. Therefore, many inappropriate referrals can be made, creating a huge caseload on popular disciplines such as physiotherapy.

The first contact of the patient should be someone who has the necessary skills to assess the patient fully, the authority to make the necessary referrals and the ability to act as a gatekeeper for other services. For example, the clinician (whether specialist nurse, neurologist or rehabilitation physician) should be able to assess the gait, orthoses, communication, and so on in order to be able to determine if further referral for a more specialist opinion is worthwhile. This highly skilled specialist would be able to find the time to play this role if freed from the model of routine annual appointments. The savings made in the reduction of the inappropriate referrals could be huge and would justify the cost of having such a specialist as the first contact for the patient.

Patients with Parkinson's disease or epilepsy are unique as alterations of drug types or dosage is the usual intervention needed. Specialist nurses for these disorders have an extensive knowledge about the medications used and are in a good position to provide expert advice regarding routine drug therapy. The specialist nurse can contact the neurologist if difficulties arise.

Management of rapidly progressive neurological disorders such as motor neurone disease or Duchenne muscular dystrophy (DMD) is very complex, with medical and therapy efforts often integrated with palliative care, including psychological and social support. An explicit care pathway should be formulated to ensure adequate support is available to all patients. Patients with rapidly progressive neurological disorders need regular reviews by clinicians specialised in their disorder, with a timely access to other services when needed.

Ataxia in multiple sclerosis

A 43-year-old woman with a 15 year history of primary progressive multiple sclerosis was referred by her GP because of worsening gait and hand function plus visual problems. The patient reported several falls in- and outdoors in the previous few months. The patient's disorder manifested mainly with spastic paraparesis and ataxia, which was worse in the right side. Clinically, the main difference noted since her last appointment was worsening of her ataxia, with intention tremors, dysmetria and significant nystagmus. Several options to tackle her worsening ataxia were discussed with her.

Comments

Ataxia is a common neurological impairment that is rarely present in isolation. In its severe form, it affects not only mobility, posture and hand function but also vision, speech and swallowing (Table 4.1).

Ataxia presents the patient and clinicians with a complex management challenge. Common causes of ataxia such as multiple sclerosis and hereditary ataxias are often progressive and associated with other neurological impairments such as pyramidal weakness and sensory loss. Consequently, careful assessment of the patient is paramount to determine the impact of the neurological impairments on the functional abilities of the patient and, more importantly, to identify the compensatory mechanisms that the patient adopts to improve posture, gait or hand function. Some of these compensatory postures or movements are counterproductive in the long term and

Table 4.1. Impairment, disability and management options for ataxia

Impairment	Functional loss	Possible management strategies
Ataxia of lower limbs	Affects gait, transfers; causes falls	Physiotherapy, mobility aids, environmental adaptations
Truncal ataxia	Poor posture; pain; affects transfers	Physiotherapy, appropriate seating system, environmental adaptations
Upper limb tremors	Impairs hand function	Equipment, adaptations, surgical intervention (deep brain stimulation)
Nystagmus, oscillopsia	Visual impairment	Visual aids (prisms), medications sensory rehabilitation
Dysarthria	Communication impairment	Speech therapy, communication aids

minimizing their impact should be a part of the patient rehabilitation programme.

In its mild and early stage, ataxia can affect mainly the patient's gait and hand function. Physiotherapy is usually helpful at that stage, teaching the patient several balance exercises and occasionally providing the patient with a walking aid. Mobility aids have both advantages and disadvantages. They definitely help the patient's gait by providing support. Some patients report that the main advantage of the walking stick is that people in crowded open spaces give them more room or that people do not think that they are drunk. Some image-conscious patients reject walking aids. There is no consensus among therapists about the balance between the benefits of walking aids and their disadvantages, such as their effects on upper limbs, reduced muscle strength and mass in the lower limbs and the reduction in weight bearing of the contralateral leg.

Hand function can be significantly affected by the mildest of intention tremors or dysmetria. There is no evidence that hand therapy is effective. However, occupational therapists can help patients by providing equipment or adaptations to everyday activities.

The priority in the management of moderately severe ataxia is to improve the stability of the trunk and the proximal joints. Supportive seating systems will not only improve posture but also help upper limb function by stabilising the trunk. Most patients report improvement in non-specific discomfort or back pain occasionally associated with truncal ataxia once they have an appropriate seating system. There is a thin line between providing adequate support and restricting the patient's movement completely, causing pain and discomfort.

Some patients report improvement in truncal ataxia by wearing pressure garments. The rational of using the garment is to increase the sensory feedback, which will subsequently enable the patient to exert more control over their trunk posture. The same garments could be used in upper limbs to improve upper limb function, not only in ataxia but also for other movement disorders such as athetosis.

As many patients will have associated muscle spasticity, great attention should be paid to the management strategies to treat high muscle tone. High muscle tone can allow some patients to improve their stability, and aggressive management of spasticity, with a subsequent reduction of muscle tone, may worsen posture or limb function.

Among a mixed group of patients with ataxia, 28% will have double vision, 16% will have reduction of visual acuity and 5% will have oscillopsia. Oscillopsia is a very unpleasant problem characterised by jumping or blurring of the external world owing to poor stabilisation of the retinal images. It happens even when the head is stable. A few reports have suggested that gabapentin reduces nystagmus. Retrobulbar or intramuscular botulinum toxin can reduce nystagmus or oscillopsia but it can affect the conjugate eye movements, leading to diplopia or ptosis. Prisms could be tried if the nystagmus is less severe in one direction. Despite some positive reports of surgery for congenital nystagmus, surgery is not often successful in the management of ataxic eye movements.

Drug management of ataxia is rarely effective. Several medications such as isonizide, gabapentin, carbamazepine, primidone and clonazepam have been reported to improve ataxia to some extent. None proved effective in a randomised, controlled trial. Beta blockers, which are very effective in managing essential tremors, are not useful in treating intention tremors secondary to ataxia. Occasionally, patients have report some improvement in their stability when they are prescribed drugs such as gabapentin, which was commenced to tackle a different clinical problem such as neuropathic pain. It is very difficult to ascertain if the reported improvement was linked to reduction of pain or was a genuine positive impact of the drug on the ataxia.

Stereotactic deep brain stimulation can be appropriate for a small number of patients. The technique can target different areas in the brain to manage different clinical problems (Table 4.2) and is a well-established and effective treatment option for movement disorders in Parkinson's disease. This is mainly because of the relatively localised pathology in this disorder. In multiple sclerosis there is a heterogenous distribution of lesions in several anatomical locations. Consequently, the outcome of deep brain stimulation is less predictable. Thalamic deep brain stimulation can mainly help with intention tremors. It will not affect other ataxic manifestations such as

Table 4.2. Usual targets for deep brain stimulation

Neurological condition	Target area
Parkinson's disease	Subthalamic nucleus
Dystonia	Globus pallidus internus
Intention tremors (e.g. in multiple sclerosis)	Thalamus

dysemetria or, more importantly, truncal ataxia. A robust selection process and clear explanation to the patient about what they should expect from the procedure is extremely important. Deep brain stimulation is not without risks and a benefit/risk assessment must be discussed with the patient.

Further reading

Berk, C., Carr, J., Sinden, M., Marzke, J., Honey, C. R. (2002). Thalamic deep brain stimulation for the treatment of tremor due to multiple sclerosis: a prospective study of tremor and quality of life. *J Neurosurg* **97**, 815–820.

Kirker, S. (2001). Oscillopsia. *Adv clin Neurosci Rehabil* **1**, 22–23.

Perlman, S. L. (2000). Cerebellar Ataxia. *Curr Treat Option Neurol* **2**, 215–224.

Psychiatric manifestations in Huntington's disease

A 44-year-old man with Huntington's disease was referred to the acute hospital by his GP. The patient has been self-neglecting for months. Because of his anxiety, he did not leave his house for weeks and he also developed paranoid delusions about his family and neighbours.

Comments

Huntington's disease is an autosomal dominant neurological degenerative disorder. In the western world, it has a population prevalence of 4–10 cases per 100 000. There are some exceptions to this generally constant prevalence, with countries such as Finland and Japan reporting much lower prevalence. This is probably because of the relative isolation of the population in these countries. Most patients present in their thirties and the median age of death is around 55.

The description made by George Huntington in his seminal paper in 1872 still stands true today. He described the triad of a movement disorder, cognitive impairment and significant psychiatric and behavioural manifestations. George Huntington observed the full penetration of the defected gene, as he was able to review the notes on affected families managed by his father and grandfather who were physicians in the same practice. In the following 100 years, and as Huntington's disease became traditionally managed mainly by neurologists, significant interest was paid to the motor and movement impairment, with relatively less emphasis on the cognitive and psychiatric manifestations. Most of the observational and therapeutic trials were directed at the movement disorder. This approach was unjustified as the psychiatric and behavioural difficulties are not only the presenting features in many cases but they also present the main challenges facing carers and treating clinicians throughout the course of the disease.

Physical manifestations of the disease vary. However, chorea is the most common movement disorder and can be very disabling and problematic in the middle and late stages of the disease. Other movement disorders such as dystonia, bradykinesia and akathesia are not uncommon. Patients can also have problems with their swallowing and that, in conjunction with an increased calorie requirement resulting from the continuous and excessive movements, may lead to a considerable weight loss and cachexia. Nutrition via a gastrostomy tube is occasionally needed. Incontinence is common in the late stages and is mainly a consequence of worsening dementia.

Chorea has traditionally been the focus of pharmacological management. This is certainly appropriate in patients with severe chorea and subsequent problems with mobility, swallowing or high risk of injury. Dopamine antagonists such as chlorpromazine or tetrabenazine are usually effective in reducing the intensity and energy requirements of the patients. These medications can, however, worsen other movement disorders such as dystonia or bradykinesia. They can also reduce cognitive function further. The need for these drugs should be assessed carefully as they probably have very limited value in the early and middle stages of the disease.

The psychiatric and behavioural manifestations of Huntington's disease are very common and diverse. Almost 98% of patients will be affected by a significant psychiatric illness at some stage. In most cases, the psychiatric manifestations are non-specific, and patients present with a combination of anxiety symptoms such as obsessive–compulsive disorders and agitation. Apathy and depression are also common. Psychotic symptoms and disinhibition seem to affect younger patients in the early stages of their illness and patients affected in this way usually have a significantly poorer prognosis.

The first manifestations of Huntington's disease in 80% of patients are psychiatric or behavioural. This is an important observation especially now that several trials are targeting this group of patients with very early disease to try to stop or delay the development of symptoms using experimental pharmacological or genetic methods. In 1983, the gene defective in Huntington's disease was localised to chromosome four, and 10 years later the gene was identified. A simple laboratory test is now available for any patient at risk of Huntington's disease. As no effective treatment to delay or alter the nature of the disease exists, the test should only be taken after appropriate genetic counselling.

The toxic effect of the abnormal protein (huntingtin) expressed by the faulty gene is evident in the basal ganglia, with subsequent atrophy of the striatal structures. Several cortical and subcortical areas show similar degenerative changes as the disease progresses. This anatomical distribution explains most of the motor and cognitive manifestations of Huntington's disease. The pathophysiology of the variable psychiatric symptoms is poorly understood.

The impact of the cognitive, psychiatric and behavioural impairments on both patients and their carers cannot be underestimated. The cognitive difficulties are usually slowly progressive but eventually present with a clinical picture that is consistent with the diagnosis of subcortical dementia, with predominant attention difficulties and impairment of higher executive function (frontal lobe syndrome). The clinical picture of the subcortical dementia can explain some of the psychiatric and behavioural problems such as apathy and personality changes. More serious and disabling psychiatric impairments can present in the early stages of the disease before the onset of the full-blown dementia syndrome. These psychiatric symptoms are often very distressing for the patients and carers.

With the complex presentation of Huntington's disease, management pathways should contain a wide neuropsychiatric perspective and encourage utilisation of the modern neuropsychological interventions available. Such an approach would best suit the needs of the patients and carers throughout the course of the disease.

Reference

Huntington, G. (1872). On chorea. *Med Surg Reporter* **26**, 317–321. (Republished in *Adv Neurolol* (1973) **1**, 33–35.)

Further reading

Paulsen, J. S., Ready, R. E., Hamilton, J. M., Mega, M. S., Cummings, J. L. (2001). Neuropsychiatric aspects of Huntington's disease. *J Neurol Neurosurg Psychiatry* **71**, 310–314.

Tost, H., Wendt, C. S., Schmitt, A., Heinz, A., Braus, D. F. (2004). Huntington's disease: phenomenological diversity of a neuropsychiatric condition that challenges traditional concepts in neurology and psychiatry. *Am J Psychiatry* **161**, 28–34.

The adult patient with Duchenne muscular dystrophy

A referral letter was received from the paediatric service asking to transfer a 16-year-old with DMD to the adult neurological rehabilitation service. The patient had no current active medical problems. He had an S-shape scoliosis managed surgically when he was 12. The patient was obese and wheelchair dependent and using an indoors–outdoors powered wheelchair. He was on no regular medications. He has planned to do a graphic design course in college.

Comments

Thanks to the advances in the management of the respiratory and cardiac complications of DMD, the average age of death has increased to 25 years. Therefore, dealing with DMD as a mainly child health disorder is unjustified. Most patients with DMD are transferred to adult services, where they are expected to receive optimum care for their complex needs.

This dystrophy is inherited as an X-recessive disorder affecting 1 in 3000 male births. In 1986, researchers managed to pinpoint the affected gene in the X chromosome of such patients. The gene is responsible for the production of a large protein known as **dystrophin**. Complete failure to produce this protein from the defective gene is the main pathology in DMD, leading to proliferation of fatty and connective tissues in the muscular structure and resulting in the classic **pseudohypertrophy** of the large muscles in the early stages of the disease.

By the time the patient is transferred to the adult services, he is invariably wheelchair dependent. Mild learning disability is associated with DMD; however, most patients have normal or higher than average intelligence. Leaving school and the paediatric health services can be unsettling for many patients and many services adopt the model of formal joint clinics between the paediatric and adult teams to facilitate the patient's transfer and to help the adult team to identify any active issues that need addressing in the early stages of dealing with the patient.

Regular physiotherapy is not usually needed at that stage; however, efforts should continue to provide mechanical correction of the muscular dysfunction in order to maintain satisfactory posture and compensate for muscle weakness. Wheelchair provision is of paramount importance. Most patients will need special seating systems because of their poor truncal and neck control. A powered wheelchair can reduce the patient's dependence.

Another important member of the multidisciplinary team is the nutritionist. Many patients with DMD are either obese or malnourished. Both conditions can be very detrimental for the patient, with obesity worsening respiratory function and mobility on the one hand and malnourishment reducing immunity and increasing the risk of osteoporosis on the other.

Scoliosis is almost universal in such patients. During childhood, it is usually monitored and surgical management considered if the Cobb's angle reaches 30–40 degrees. Scoliosis should be optimally managed as it is one of the reasons for worsening respiratory function in the late stages. Surgical management should also be planned before the respiratory function deteriorates to an extent that would be an unacceptable risk for an operation.

Respiratory failure is by far the most common cause of death in DMD. The patient's ineffective cough and decreased ventilation lead to recurrent problems with pneumonia, atlectasis and respiratory insufficiency. The patient should receive pneumococcal vaccination and yearly influenza vaccine and should have a respiratory review at least twice a year to detect the earliest signs of deterioration in respiratory function.

During these reviews, pulse oxymetry, forced vital capacity, forced expiratory volume in the first second, maximal mid-expiratory flow rate and peak cough flow should be measured. During the assessment, other causes of respiratory dysfunction, such as obstructive sleep apnoea or reflux oesophagitis, should be excluded.

Many measures can be recommended to slow down the deterioration of respiratory function. Maintaining airway clearance can be achieved either manually or mechanically using modern assisted-cough technologies. Respiratory muscle training should also be an integral part of the routine management of the patient.

Commencement of non-invasive nocturnal ventilation should be strongly recommended to the patients when indicated. Some authors believe that this method of management should only be started after the patient has had a full polysomnography study. Other authors would start non-invasive ventilation if pulse oxymetry showed persistent nocturnal hypoventilation. As the respiratory function deteriorates further, most patients will need daytime non-invasive ventilation as well.

As the disease progresses, the contentious issues of invasive ventilation arise. The patient's quality of life should be a matter for only the patient to decide. The option of invasive ventilation via a tracheostomy should be discussed frankly with the patient and his family, explaining the benefits and the potential problems such as effects on speech.

Management of the respiratory complications of DMD should ideally be the responsibility of a respiratory physician with interest and experience in dealing with the condition. Plans for hospital admission for the management of respiratory complications should be in place and a link with a hospital physician identified.

Cardiac problems are also universal in these patients, but only 30–40% will be symptomatic. Patients should see a cardiologist with an interest in DMD. An annual echocardiogram and electrocardiogram are standard practice for patients with DMD. Cardiac complications such as cardiac failure and arrhythmias are particularly apparent, leading to 10–20% of deaths in these patients.

Most of adults with DMD continue to live with their parents. Every effort should be made to increase their independence at home using different equipment and aids. Many patients find environmental control systems helpful. Additional home care or respite should be discussed with the patient and family.

Further reading

American Thoracic Society (2004). Consensus statement: respiratory care of the patient with Duchenne muscle dystrophy. *Am J Resp Crit Care Med* **170**, 456–465.

Bach, J., Alba, A., Pilkington, L. A., Lee, M. (1981). Long-term rehabilitation in advanced stage of childhood onset, rapidly progressive muscular dystrophy. *Arch Phys Med Rehabil* **62**, 328–331.

LaPrade, R. F., Rowe, D. E. (1992). The operative treatment of scoliosis in Duchenne muscular dystrophy. *Orthop Rev* **21**, 39–45.

Recurrent aspiration in a patient with Parkinson's disease

A 57-year-old man with a 12-year history of Parkinson's disease was admitted to hospital for the management of pneumonia. For the previous six months, the patient had suffered from recurrent chest infections. Aspiration was suspected as a cause of the chest infections but swallowing assessments performed on two separate occasions showed a satisfactory swallow. Clinically, the patient was immobile and wheelchair dependent. His posture was poor and a headrest was attached to his wheelchair as his neck control was severely affected. The patient also had impaired hand function and was dependent on his carers for feeding.

Comments

A safe and efficient swallowing function is dependent upon the fine coordination of many small muscles in the mouth and throat. These muscles are controlled by a complex neurological network that acts at both voluntary and involuntary levels. Impairment of higher cerebral control, brainstem function, cranial nerves or the local muscular functions can disturb this finely tuned mechanism and lead to an increased risk of aspiration.

The swallowing process can be divided into two main stages. The first is the oral preparation, which reduces food to a suitable consistency and provides the pleasure of eating. This stage involves seeing and smelling the food, which stimulates the flow of saliva in preparation for receiving the bolus. The food is chewed, mixed with saliva and is pulled together by the tongue into a single ball (bolus) in preparation to be swallowed. The oral stage of the swallow is a voluntary process and is under cortical control.

The pharyngeal stage of the swallow is triggered when the bolus reaches the anterior faucial arches. This is the involuntary stage of the swallow function and is controlled by centres located in the medulla. The processes of the pharyngeal stage are elevation of the larynx and closure of the vocal cords. The elevation of the larynx pulls open the oesophageal sphincter, allowing the epiglottis to fold over and cover it; the bolus can then fall into the vallecula directly down the oesophagus.

Food aspiration can take place before, during or after swallowing and can result from any malfunction of such a finely synchronised mechanism. Aspiration before the swallow can result from either a reduced tongue movement or a delayed or absent triggering of the swallow reflex. Aspiration during the swallow results from a reduced laryngeal closure, while aspiration after the swallow occurs when food material left in the pyriform sinuses overflows into the airway.

Clinically, many signs can act as red flags for swallowing problems (Table 4.3). During routine clinical assessments, these indicators should be documented and monitored and a referral to a speech and language therapist should be arranged for a formal swallowing assessment if swallowing impairment is suspected.

Swallowing assessment is a clinically subjective method to establish the safety and efficiency of the swallowing process. For patients who have a clearly unsafe swallowing mechanisim, non-oral feeding is recommended. Feeding via a nasogastric tube is usually used for short periods and then the patient is reviewed regularly. If the swallowing impairment is deemed to be permanent or may take a long time to recover, a robust feeding method is established such as a percutaneous endoscopic gastrostomy tube. Many patients will, however, have impaired swallowing but can increase the efficency and safety of the process by adopting several strategies (Table 4.4).

Patients with swallowing disorders are at risk of nutritional deficiencies. Many patients with swallowing disorders may also suffer from cognitive or communication impairments and so can be unable to perceive or communicate their symptoms or basic needs, which might be as basic as thirst

Table 4.3. Red flags for swallowing impairment

Reduced appetite
Weight loss
Taking a long time to finish meals
Inability to finish meals
Evidence of food/drink on clothing
Drooling
Inability to manage own saliva
Inability to take food from the fork or spoon
Poor chewing pattern and control in the mouth

Table 4.4. Common strategies used to increase the safety of swallowing

Targeted area	Strategies
General	Make sure the patient is alert
	Discourage talking while eating
	Try to position plates so the patient can see them
	Encourage the patient to eat slowly
	Wait till the patient has swallow twice
	If the patient can feed himself, encourage it with supervision
	Suggest small frequent meals
Posture	The patient should sit upright when eating
	Patient should stay sitting for 20 minutes after meals
	The chin should be forward and slightly tilted downwards while eating
Food consistency	Avoid sticky consistency (e.g. toffees) or food with mixed consistency (e.g. vegetable soup, grapes)
	Thickened fluids and liquidised diets (purées) are the easiest to swallow

or hunger. Hence nutritional deficiencies and/or dehydration are not uncommon in this group of patients. Malnutrition should be recognised and managed appropriately as it can lead to worsening of the overall clinical situation, increasing risk of infections and delaying wound healing or recovery in general. Dehydration can lead to several complications and even mild dehydration increases the risk of several significant complications such as electrolyte imbalance or renal impairment. Hyperviscosity resulting from dehydration is an important precipitating factor for thromboembolic complications.

The administration of drugs can be a major problem in patients with a swallow disorder. Some types of tablet lend themselves to being crushed and dispersed in thickened water or may also be available in liquid form. Some capsules can be emptied out and mixed with a suitable consistency, for example yoghurt. Granules can be mixed with food as for capsule contents.

It is of paramount importance to emphasise to patients the limitations of the clinical swallowing assessment, including the more invasive tests to evaluate swallowing such as video fluoroscopy. All these tests provide a snapshot of the patient, reflecting the ability to swallow in a more or less artificial enviroment such as the hospital or clinic. Once the patient is back in the community, he/she will be vulnerable to factors such as minor illnesses, fatigue or simply wanting the odd food that is difficult to swallow. All these will increase the patient's vulnerability to aspiration; so it is not uncommon to find patients passing their clinic swallowing assessment and then suffering from recurrent chest infections secondary to aspiration. A robust review of these patients will be needed, preferably at home. Their posture, food types and consistency and the skills of all their carers should all be documented, with explicit recommendations according to the findings. Some therapists recommend a sliding scale for their patients, so the patient can have a safer consistency of food if the carers feel that he/she is tired or is suffering from a minor illness.

Further reading

Corcoran, L. (2005). Nutrition and hydration tips for stroke patients with dysphagia. *Nurs Times* **101**, 24–27.

Smithard, D. G., O'Neill, P. A., Park, C., *et al.* (1998). Can bedside assessment reliably exclude aspiration following acute stroke? *Age Ageing* **27**, 99–106.

Volonte, M. A., Porta, M., Gomi, G. (2002). Clinical assessment of dysphagia in early phases of Parkinson's disease. *Neurol Sci Suppl* **2A**, S121–S122.

5

Medical complications of immobility

The effects of prolonged bed rest are well documented, with cardiovascular, respiratory, metabolic and musculoskeletal changes taking place within days of the onset of immobility. In immobile, neurologically impaired patients, several factors can add to the complexity of the situation and put the patient at even higher risk of complications. Lower limb paralysis, sensory loss, autonomic dysfunction and respiratory impairment are not uncommon in neurological disorders and all can lead to immobility.

Assessment of the immobile patient can be difficult, as many of them will need a hoist for transfers to enable the clinician to carry out a thorough examination. Special care should be taken on examining the vulnerable skin areas, the range of movements of large joints and the cardiac and respiratory systems. Review of the patient's transfers, sleeping and seating systems is also mandatory.

A few clinical syndromes, such as thromboembolism and pressure ulcers, stand out as the most serious complications of immobility. However, despite the high profile of these problems, there are still many questions and controversies regarding the best way to prevent and manage them effectively.

Thromboembolism

A 34-year-old man was admitted to the rehabilitation ward with a diagnosis of Guillain–Barré syndrome. The onset five weeks previous was with sudden onset of ascending flaccid paralysis a week after a diarrhoeal illness. The paralysis affected the respiratory and bulbar muscles and the patient required artificially ventilation for 16 days. On admission, the patient was only receiving injections of low-molecular-weight heparin (Enoxaparin, 40 mg) for thromboprophylaxis.

Despite intensive physiotherapy for four months, the patient's physical recovery was limited. He regained upper limb and sphincteric functions but remained wheelchair dependent. He could transfer independently but could only stand and take a few steps if supported by therapists. Clinically, he had considerable wasting of the muscles of his lower limbs, with flaccid paralysis; muscle power was 3/5 in most muscle groups. The patient also had considerable sensory ataxia.

On the last ward round before discharge, the patient asked about his Enoxaparin injections. He wanted to know for how long these would continue.

Comments

Immobility is a major risk factor for venous thromboembolism and neurological diseases with extremity paresis account for 7% of all these events. The literature has clearly shown the value of prophylactic anticoagulation in reducing the risk of venous thromboembolism in patients admitted to hospital for surgical and medical management of conditions such as hip fractures, cardiac failure or respiratory failure. Duration of anticoagulation is usually one or two weeks in order to match the usual duration of hospitalisation and immobility among these patients.

Patients who are immobile because of neurological impairments present a unique problem as they tend to be immobile for prolonged periods of time and a significant number never regain independent mobility. In conditions that lead to acute deterioration of mobility (e.g. acute spinal cord injury and Guillain–Barré syndrome), thromboprophylaxis is strongly recommended as thromboembolic complications are extremely common. Duration of anticoagulation is less straightforward as most of these patients remain immobile for long periods. The only clear guidelines deal with acute spinal cord injury, as this group of patients has been extensively studied. The incidence of venous thromboembolism in spinal cord injuries decreases dramatically after the first four months to a level similar to that of the general population. Therefore, patients with acute spinal cord injuries should receive thromboprophylaxis for only four months even if they remain immobile following that period.

The question of whether a general principle for any immobile neurologically impaired patient can be based on the observations in the chronic phase of spinal cord injury depends on the mechanism by which risk of venous thromboembolism reduces in this group once the acute phase has passed. Two main mechanisms have been suggested: vascular atrophy and muscular spasticity.

The difficulty with the patient described in the case study above is that he will never develop muscle spasticity as Guillain–Barré syndrome is an ascending neuropathy. However, vascular changes alone might provide adequate protection and justify discontinuation of prophylactic measures when these changes are established.

The vascular changes in the paralysed lower limbs are well documented. There is a generalised atrophy of the arteries and reduced blood flow to the paralysed lower limbs, which represents adaptations to a lower oxygen demand. This process is usually well established within six weeks of onset of the lower limb paralysis and leads to reduced blood flow in the calf veins, with shrinkage in vein size and dispensability. This process will then reduce the stasis and pooling of blood that usually happens after sudden onset of paralysis and is the major factor for the development of venous thromboembolism.

There is circumstantial evidence for a low risk of venous thromboembolism in patients who are immobile over a long period whether their lower limb paralysis is spastic or not. For example, disabling conditions that are not associated with neurological disorders such as severe rheumatoid arthritis do not seem to be prone to venous thrombosis despite causing immobility. Patients suffering strokes have the highest risk of venous thromboembolism in the first two to four weeks despite spasticity only occurring in a minority of patients following a stroke.

Venous thromboembolism is a multi causal condition with different risk factors, such as age, immobility and genetic factors. They all act to reduce the patient's threshold for developing a deep vein thrombosis. It is clear from the literature that the acute period of immobility is the most dangerous. It is simplistic to assume that either muscle spasticity or vascular changes are the only factors reducing the risk of thromboembolism in the long term. In chronically immobile patients, several factors interact to increase the risk again. These factors should be considered in the clinical setting to guide decisions to continue or to stop any thromboprophylactic strategies such as anticoagulant use. However, in the absence of any guidance regarding an optimal duration for prophylactic anticoagulation, the robust thromboprophylaxis guidelines used in spinal injuries could be extrapolated to other neurological conditions. This would suggest that it is safe to discontinue thromboprophylaxis four months following the acute onset of immobility in a young patient with no added risk factor for venous thromboembolism other than immobility. The patient in the case study here should be counselled that the risk of venous thromboembolism will not be eliminated and his views about the management should be considered.

Greater Manchester Neurorehabilitation Network has guidelines for thromboprophylaxis of the immobile neurologically impaired patients (Figure 5.1).

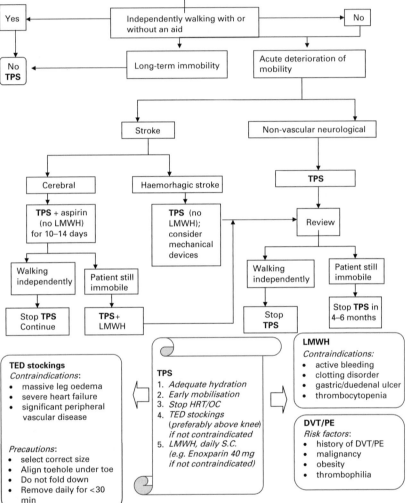

Figure 5.1. Guidelines for thromboprophylaxis strategy (TPS) from the Greater Manchester Neurorehabilitation Network. TED, thromboembolism deterrent; LMWH, low-molecular-weight heparin; DVT, deep vein thrombosis; PE, pulmonary embolism; s.c., subcutaneous injection; HRT/OC, hormone replacement therapy/oral contraceptives. (From Gaber, T. (2006). *Disabil Rehabil* 28, 1413–1416. www.informaworld.com.)

Further reading

Consensus Conference on Deep Venous Thrombosis in Spinal Cord Injury (1999). Summary and recommendations. *Chest* **102**(suppl), 6335.

Gaber, T. A. (2005). Significant reduction of the risk of venous thromboembolism in all long term immobile patients a few months after onset of immobility. *Med Hypoth* **64**, 1173–1176.

Turpie, A. G., Chin, B. S., Lip, G. Y. l. (2002). ABC of antithrombotic therapy. Venous thromboembolism: pathophysiology, clinical features and prevention. *BMJ* **325**, 887–890.

Osteoporosis

After two incidents of fracture neck of femur following falls in the neurorehabilitation unit, staff suggested screening all inpatients for osteoporosis or to provide bone prophylaxis for all. No guidelines were found and further opinion was sought.

Comments

The pathogenesis of immobility-induced osteoporosis is not fully understood. It is generally accepted that reduction of mechanical loading secondary to either lessening tendon pull of the attaching trabecular bones or reduced gravitational force leads to demineralisation. This process is probably the main reason for the low bone mass of the sedentary population with generally reduced habitual activities.

Sudden onset of immobility in neurological paralysis leads to rapid loss of bone in the paralysed region of the body mainly caused by reduced osteoblastic activity. Despite normal serum calcium, immobilised patients are hypercalciuric with increased calcium urinary secretion peaking four to five weeks after the onset of immobility and continuing for up to a year afterwards. It is important to appreciate this fact, as even when some patients develop hypercalcaemia in the acute phase after immobility, their total body calcium balance is negative.

Osteoporosis is a multifactorial disorder. Immobility often acts in conjunction with other factors such as old age in stroke patients or steroid intake during relapses in patients with multiple sclerosis. Many patients will already have low bone mass before the onset of the neurological insult, and the

Table 5.1. Significance of T and Z scores

Score	Use	Derivation
T	Diagnosis of osteopenia and osteoporosis	$\dfrac{\text{Measured BMD} - \text{Young adult mean BMD}}{\text{Young adult standard deviation}}$
Z	Comparison of BMD with age-matched normal population	$\dfrac{\text{Measured BMD} - \text{Age-matched mean BMD}}{\text{Age-matched standard deviation}}$

BMD, bone mineral density.

Table 5.2. Osteopenia and osteoporosis from the T score

	Definition
Osteopenia	BMD 1–2.5 SD below the young adult mean value
Osteoporosis	BMD $\geq$2.5 SD below the young adult mean value

BMD, bone mineral density; SD, standard deviation.

immobility will increase the severity of the osteoporosis. In a mixed group of patients admitted to a rehabilitation unit, 60% had osteoporosis.

Bone mass can be assessed by different methods, for example quantitative ultrasound or computer axial tomography. However, dual-energy X-ray absorptometry (DXA) remains the gold standard for bone mass measurement. This technique usually expresses the bone mass measurements as Z and T scores (Table 5.1) in three main body sites: neck of femur, lumbar spine and lower forearm bilaterally. It enables the clinician to diagnose either osteopenia or osteoporosis using the T scores (Table 5.2).

Sudden or long-term immobility is not among the recommended indications for DEXA measurement suggested by the Royal College of Physicians (Table 5.3). Therefore, it is difficult to justify mass screening of immobilised patients with neurological impairment if they do not have one of the listed concurrent pathologies. Routine bone prophylaxis is inappropriate in the absence of a DEXA measurements baseline.

Many clinicians argue against this rational, citing many studies in patients with spinal injuries or strokes that clearly show high incidence of osteoporosis in this group. Such patients might be more susceptible to low-impact trauma such as falls, leading to high risk of bone fractures especially in vulnerable areas such as hips and wrists. Such fractures might have a catastrophic effect on the patient's rehabilitation programme and its ultimate outcome.

Table 5.3. Royal College of Physicians indications for assessment by dual-energy x-ray absorptometry

Radiographic evidence of osteopenia or osteporosis
Loss of height, thoracic kyphosis
Previous fragility fracture
Prolonged corticosteroid therapy
Premature menopause
Prolonged secondary amenorrhoea
Primary hypogonadism
Chronic disorders associated with osteoporosis (e.g. malabsorption)
Maternal history of hip fracture
Low body mass index ($< 19 \, \text{kg/m}^2$)

Other clinicians feel that mass screening is unjustified as most patients will regain mobility and build up their bone mass again; consequently, bone prophylaxis will probably not be beneficial as the period of high risk is relatively short. If the patient never regains independent mobility, risk of trauma is minimal, making it difficult to evaluate cost/benefit balance. Unfortunately, such issues have never been examined and no data are available to guide clinicians regarding the cost-effectiveness of routine screening.

Some steps could be taken to minimise the risk of osteoporosis during rehabilitation. Standing on a tilt table or standing frame as soon as possible might help patients maintain bone mass. The same methods could be implemented with wheelchair-dependent patients in the community. Resistant exercises would also be very useful to ensure that the bones receive regular muscle pull.

Patients who present with immobility hypercalcaemia should receive a biphosphonate as a first line of management. Biphosphonates will reverse the original pathology, increasing osteoblastic activity and subsequently reducing the rate of calcium release from the bones. This should reduce hypercalcaemia and hypercalciuria and also help to reduce the risk of renal stones, which patients are predisposed to especially with long-term catheterisation.

Pamidronate is a potent agent reducing bone resorption. It could be particularly useful in immobility-induced hypercalcaemia as it is usually given intravenously in a single dose, with its effects lasting for months. In a recent report, pamidronate failed to preserve bone density two years after spinal cord injury despite its initial success in reducing bone resorption in the immediate aftermath of the spinal injury.

The main goal for the treatment of osteoporosis is to prevent the first low-impact bone fracture. Patients admitted for rehabilitation are usually very varied, with different ages, medical conditions, drug histories and levels of mobility. A compromise between the extremes of mass screening or doing nothing seems the best approach to such a difficult issue. Stratification of patients based on their risk factors for osteoporosis and their general risk of falls might identify a group with the highest risk of fracture. If a diagnosis of osteoporosis is made, management should be with both medical intervention and other methods to minimise the risk of fractures, such as the use of hip protectors or more supportive mobility aids.

Further reading

Bauman, W. A., Wecht, J. M., Kirshblum, S., *et al.* (2005). Effect of pamidronate administration in bone in patients with acute spinal cord injury. *J Rehabil Res Dev* **42**, 305–314.

Hain, S. F. (2006). DXA scanning for osteporosis. *Clin Med* **6**, 254–258.

Liu, M., Tsuji, T., Higuchi, Y., *et al.* (1999). Osteoporosis in hemiplegic stroke patients as studied with dual-energy X-ray absorptometry. *Am J Phys Med Rehabil* **80**, 1213–1226.

Pressure sores

A 52-year-old woman with a 28 year history of multiple sclerosis developed a deep sacral and a left heel pressure sore. The patient was immobile because of a combination of spastic paraplegia and ataxia. Clinically both pressure sores extended deep into the muscle with deep necrotic tissue in the bed of the sore.

Comments

Almost all pressure sores are caused by unrelieved pressure on soft tissues between a bone and a hard surface such as a bed or a trolley. Such pressure will interrupt the local microcirculation, leading to hypoxia and subsequent necrosis. A less-known but nonetheless important factor in the development of pressure sores is the shearing or friction forces, which is crucial in patients with severe immobility such as tetraplegics. These patients are exposed to significant shearing forces during their transfers and also are unable to feel the impact of friction because of sensory impairments. Many other factors increase the risk of pressure sores, such as incontinence, cognitive impairment and nutritional deficiencies. These factors are routinely assessed when patients are admitted to hospital to stratify the risk of pressure sore development using standardised measures such as the Braden and the Waterloo Scores.

Most patients admitted to rehabilitation units are at high risk of developing pressure sores. Immobility is a crucial factor and in combination with other risk factors it puts the patient at very high risk. Such patients should have a comprehensive plan to stop pressure sores developing, including using pressure-relieving mattresses/cochins, correction of nutritional deficiencies, catheterisation for urinary incontinence and review of their seating system and methods of transfers to reduce the impact of the shearing forces.

Many patients with long-term disabilities such as spinal injuries and multiple sclerosis will have a continuing high risk as many of the risk factors are difficult to resolve. Patients should be encouraged to take some responsibility for prevention measures if possible, checking vulnerable areas regularly using a mirror and doing several pressure-relieving movements regularly while in his/her wheelchair.

Once a pressure sore is detected, several measures should be immediately implemented. Bed rest is an effective but unpopular measure for patients. Wheelchair use often puts more pressure on vulnerable areas than does bed rest as the latter distributes the body weight over a wider surface area. More frequent baths should be encouraged to try to remove necrotic tissues and reduce the risk of proliferation of colonising bacteria.

Several ways to classify and stage pressure sores have been developed to assess severity and response to treatment. **Torrance's developmental classification** is the most widely used (Table 5.4).

All risk factors for pressure sore development should be tackled simultaneously. An appropriate pressure-relieving mattress should be provided. A full medical assessment should be carried out to identify any comorbidity that could delay healing. Common medical conditions such as anaemia and hypoalbuminaemia are common and relatively easy to correct. No effort should be spared to improve the state of the cardiovascular and respiratory systems to ensure adequate oxygenation of the affected area. Lower limb spasms are a common predisposing cause of heel ulcers, and robust methods to control these spasms should be implemented.

Table 5.4. Staging of pressure sores

Stage	Features
1	Blanching hyperaemia
2	Non-blanching hyperaemia
3	Ulceration extending to the dermis
4	Ulceration extending to the subcutaneous fat
5	Infective necrosis penetrating to the deep fascia

Table 5.5. Methods used for wound debridement

Method	Comment
Moist wound healing dressings	Hydrocolloids and hydrogels promote debridement by rehydrating and softening dead tissues; the simple and popular debridement method
Wound irrigation	Using saline or water either as a pressure spray or a bath
Cadexomers	Debrides ulcers by absorbing fluid and debris and delivering a healing agent like *iodine* to the sore surface
Enzymatic debridement	Such as streptokinase; loosing popularity now because of lack of evidence of effectiveness
Larvae therapy	Using *maggot larvae*, which can ingest the necrotic tissues and produce bactericidal enzymes
Surgical debridement	Can be undertaken at the bedside or in the theatre; *hydrocolloid dressing* is usually used initially to soften the tissues before debridement.

Removal of dead necrotic tissues is the priority when managing the pressure sore locally. A variety of methods are available for removal of dead tissue (Table 5.5). The initial assessment is crucial as some pressure sores are so extensive and the necrotic process is too advanced to waste valuable time trying methods such as saline soaks or hydrocolloid dressings. A surgical review may not only establish the need for surgical debridement but can also explore surgical management plans to help in the long-term management of the pressure sore. One of the common problems that may need surgical intervention is the presence of a track that goes deeper into the ulcer and can complicate the healing process.

Infection commonly occurs with pressure sores and its management is often controversial. Systemic antibiotics should not be used routinely as bacterial growth is not usually associated with tissue reactions. The indications for systemic antibiotic use are the presence of septicaemia, local cellulites or the growth of a very virulent bacterial strain locally. Topical antibiotics are rarely used as they can encourage the emergence of antibiotic-resistant bacterial strains. Unpleasant odours are usually managed by an activated charcoal dressing.

Once a pressure sore is clean with no evidence of active infection, healing is a matter of good supportive management and time. In some patients with deep sores, the large surface area involved makes spontaneous healing difficult and sometimes impossible. Several methods such as plastic surgery can help. A popular method to tackle this problem is the use of **negative pressure therapy**. The technique involves applying an open-pore foam dressing to the wound, which is then sealed using a transparent adhesive drape to create a controlled closed wound environment. A negative pressure is then applied across the wound via a drainage tube embedded in the foam. Theoretically such negative pressure will increase blood flow, subsequently reducing local tissue oedema and bacterial colonisation. The negative pressure can also reduce the exudates production and encourage granulating tissues formation.

Further reading

Argenta, L. C., Morykwas M. J. (1997). Vacuum-assisted closure: a new method for wound control and treatment. Clinical experience. *Ann Plastic Surg* **38**, 563–576.

Heterotopic ossification

A 28-year-old man suffered a complete T8 spinal injury following a motorcycle accident. Five weeks after admission to the spinal injuries unit, the patient complained of pain in the left hip. Clinically, the whole left leg was swollen and painful with the hip showing significant hotness and tenderness with severe pain in passive movement. A plain radiograph showed evidence of soft tissues calcification close to the left hip articular surfaces.

Comments

Heterotopic ossification is a condition in which mature lamellar bone is formed in tissues that do not normally ossify. The term has replaced several names that used to be used to describe soft tissue ossification, such as myositis ossificans.

Heterotopic ossification is believed to result from metaplasia of the mesenchymal cells in soft tissues, with subsequent proliferation of bone-forming osteoblasts. The trigger for this cellular metaplasia is poorly understood but humeral or neural triggers are probably implicated. Alterations of sympathetic neural connections following brain or spinal injury or repetitive trauma resulting from joint manipulation might also contribute to the transformation process.

Several conditions can precipitate heterotopic ossification. The biggest risk factor is a past history of the disorder and almost all patients with such a history will go on to develop it again if exposed to a major orthopaedic procedure such as hip surgery. It also develops in 10–30% of patients with significant neurological impairments secondary to conditions such as spinal or brain injury. Patients with spinal injuries are particularly vulnerable with heterotopic ossification affecting large joints such as hips, knees, shoulders and elbows – always below the level of the neurological injury – and causing severe local pain, redness, hotness and reduced range of movement. Generalised symptoms such as fever and malaise are not uncommon in severe cases. The differential diagnoses include conditions such as deep venous thrombosis, cellulitis, joint sepsis, haematoma and bony fracture.

Laboratory tests are typically normal with the exception of alkaline phosphatase, erythrocyte sedimentation rate and C-reactive protein, which are usually moderately raised a few weeks after the onset and are good indicators of disease activity. Plain radiographs are diagnostic in clear-cut cases. In mild and early heterotopic ossification, a three-phase bone scan is a valuable tool to identify its occurrence and it also can establish maturity in advanced disease. Both CT and MRI have roles, especially for preoperative evaluation to check the extent of heterotopic ossification and its relation to blood vessels. The scans can also help to exclude other pathologies such as a calcified haematoma or tumour.

During the acute phase of heterotopic ossification, short-term rest will be needed to minimise the inflammatory process. However, it is important to continue the rehabilitation programme including mobilising the affected joint within the range of painless movement. If joint manipulation worsens pain or seems to increase the inflammatory process, it should be discontinued until the patient is able to tolerate it.

Several reports suggested the efficacy of bisphosphonates, particularly disodium etidronate, in at least halting the progression of heterotopic ossification. The standard practice is to administer disodium etidronate intravenously for three days and then orally for six months. Regular measurements of alkaline phosphatase, erythrocyte sedimentation rate and C–reactive protein is a suitable approach for monitoring the activity of heterotopic ossification.

Once disease activity has stabilised, as indicated by normal alkaline phosphatase and inflammatory markers plus a normal three-phase bone scan, a functional assessment will be needed. If heterotopic ossification does not affect the patient's functional abilities, active management will not be needed and the patient should be observed for any changes in the clinical picture.

A few patients will suffer from joint deformities that are severe enough to cause functional impairments. These patients should be assessed for suitability for surgical intervention. Surgical excision can be an effective intervention to improve the range of movement and function of the affected joint. Infection, bleeding and recurrence of heterotopic ossification are potential complications of surgery; hence, careful assessment including full explanation of potential benefits and risks to the patient is mandatory.

Several methods have been suggested to reduce the risk of heterotopic ossification recurrence after surgical excision including radiotherapy, bisphosphonates, and non-steroidal anti-inflammatory drugs (NSAIDs) especially indometacin. The use of NSAIDs is well established for prevention of heterotopic ossification after hip arthroplasty, with a Cochrane systematic review suggesting 15–20% reduction of the risk of heterotopic ossification following hip arthroplasty using NSAIDs. Whether NSAIDs have a role in the prevention of heterotopic ossification following neurological impairments is not known.

Further reading

Banovac, K., Sherman, A. L., Estores, I. M. (2004). Prevention and treatment of heterotopic ossification after spinal cord injury. *J Spinal Cord Med* **27**, 376–382.

Freebourn, T. M., Barber, D. B., Able, A. C. (1999). The treatment of immature heterotopic ossification in spinal cord injury with combination surgery, radiation therapy and NSAIDs. *Spinal Cord* **37**, 50–53.

Burd, T. A., Lowry, K. J., Anglan, J. O. (2001). Indomethacin compared with localized irradiation for the prevention of heterotopic ossification following surgical treatment of acetabular fractures. *J Bone Joint Surg Am* **83**, 1783–1788.

6

Orthotics in neurological rehabilitation

An orthotist once told me that there are thousands of types of ankle–foot orthoses (AFOs) and that he finds it difficult to keep up with all the changes taking place within his speciality. That was reassuring, as I always feel that it is unreasonable to expect rehabilitation clinicians, whether they are physicians or therapists, to be able to prescribe or even suggest the best orthotic management plan for their patients. However, I feel that it is extremely important to understand the basics of biomechanics and gait analysis to be able to assess and manage neurologically impaired patients properly. This will not only facilitate the clinical decision making when dealing with issues such as medical or surgical interventions for lower limb spasticity but can also help the treating clinician in deciding which patient will benefit most from an orthotic opinion.

If orthotists welcome referrals detailing the clinical situation, leaving the ultimate decision to the orthotist to decide the appropriate intervention, gait analysis laboratories do not. Some clinicians refer their patients for gait analysis expecting the report to provide the answers or explanation for the patient's gait impairment plus a recommendation of the appropriate management plan. This is rarely the case, as gait analysis is most valuable in establishing or refuting a particular hypothesis. It always helps when the referring clinician is able to formulate a hypothesis and then ask if the gait analysis can confirm or reject it. This approach is particularly important before offering an irreversible intervention to the patient such as Achilles tendon lengthening.

For assessment of gait in the clinic, a simpler approach could be considered. Many clinicians concentrate on the **ground reaction force** during the different stages of the gait as a simple way to evaluate the forces and moments acting on the knees and hips. I have personally found this approach extremely useful in enabling me to decide if simple interventions such as botulinum toxin injections for calf muscles, heel raise or AFOs (all moving ground reaction force backwards, creating flexion moments around the knees) are appropriate.

Secondary scoliosis

An 18-year-old man presented in the school leavers clinic with a severe cerebral palsy and moderately severe learning disability. The patient had a thoraco lumbar C-shaped scoliosis with apex pointing to the right. The plain radiograph showed a Cobb angle of 25 degrees and also showed evidence of considerable spinal rotation. The patient was using a rigid plastic thoraco lumbar orthosis and used an attendant-controlled wheelchair with a moulded seat. The lower limbs were spastic, with flexion deformities affecting the right hip, both knees and a dislocated left hip.

Comments

The definition and classification of the causes of scoliosis made more than two millennia ago by Hippocrates still stands true today. He stated that: 'There are many variations of curvatures of the spine, even in persons who are in good health, for it takes place from natural conformations (congenital and idiopathic) and from habit (functional) and the spine is liable to be bent from old age (degenerative) and pains (acquired).'

The Scoliosis Research Society has defined a medically significant scoliosis as any curve that is 10 degrees or more with or without a rotatory component. Scoliosis can be *functional or structural* (Figure 6.1). Unequal leg length, muscle spasms or poor posture are common causes of functional scoliosis, which is usually mild and reversible. Most cases of structural scoliosis are idiopathic. Idiopathic scoliosis is more common in females and the onset is usually during adolescence. Most patients present with the spine deformity with no complaint of pain or neurological dysfunction. Idiopathic scoliosis should not be confused

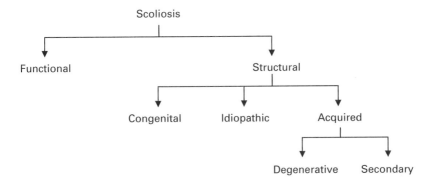

Figure 6.1 Causes of scoliosis.

with *congenital* scoliosis, which has a well-defined defect affecting the structure of the spine and is often associated with congenital neurological disorders such as neurofibromatosis or hereditary mesenchymal tissue disorders such as Ehlers-Danlos syndrome.

In a rehabilitation setting, acquired scoliosis is the most common type seen and may be associated with spinal degenerative disease, chronic back pain, osteoporosis or trauma. Acquired scoliosis is usually seen in elderly patients and mainly affects the lumbar spine.

Scoliosis secondary to congenital or acquired neurological disorders usually results from paraspinal muscle weakness in conditions leading to lower motor neurone muscle weakness, such as spinal muscle atrophy or muscle dystrophy. In upper motor neurone conditions such as cerebral palsy, a combination of muscle weakness, poor central balance control and impaired sensory feedback may contribute to the development of scoliosis. Pelvic obliquity and hip joint dislocation are also common complications of cerebral palsy and may contribute to the development of scoliosis.

Assessment of secondary scoliosis should start with a full history, with special emphasis on the primary disorder and its impact on other systems. The patient's height and leg lengths should be measured for mobile patients. Full musculoskeletal and neurological examination is mandatory, with special emphasis paid to joints stability; range of movements; and to the strength, tone and coordination of the different muscle groups including the back extensors and abdominal muscles. Cardiopulmonary assessment including vital capacity should be documented in severe disease.

Inspection of the spine should give an idea about the presence or absence of spinal rotation, with the abnormal height of the hemipelvis and shoulder indicating the severity of the lateral curve and the humping of the paraspinal muscles indicating the severity of the spinal rotation. The patient should always be asked to bend forward, as inspection of the spine in this position often enhances mild abnormalities. Reversibility of the deformity should be tested to determine if any functional component is contributing to the severity of the scoliosis.

The spinal deformity should be described in the most comprehensive and accurate way. Table 6.1 gives the standard assessment factors to describe the spinal curve. A plain radiograph should always be a part of the initial assessment or follow-up reviews. The **Cobb angle** is the standard method for objective measurement of spinal curvature. Examination of the position of the vertebral pedicles and spinous processes will indicate the severity of the spinal rotation.

Patients with secondary scoliosis provide a unique challenge, as the standard ways to manage scoliosis often fail to correct or stop the progression of the scoliosis. Problems such as hip joint dislocation, poor sitting balance, or

Table 6.1. Assessment of the scoliotic curve

Reversible or fixed
Pattern (C or S shape)
Location (thoracic, lumbar or both)
Direction of the apex
Presence or absence of spinal rotation (from radiograph)
Cobb angle: measured by dropping lines perpendicular to the endplates
    of the most tilted vertebral bodies in the curve; the Cobb angle is
    the angle at which these perpendicular lines intersect

movement disorders such as athetosis will all have an impact on the scoliosis, and addressing such problems should be included in the patient's management plan.

There is no evidence to support the use of exercise or other physical modalities in the management of scoliosis. However, a standard physiotherapy programme is essential to maintain the range of movement of joints, to reduce muscle spasticity and to improve sitting balance.

Appropriate seating and sleeping systems are essential in the management of severe scoliosis in both children and adults. A balance needs to be struck between comfort and function on one side and support and stabilisation on the other. Patients with very limited functional abilities might be able to tolerate a seating system that is very supportive, while patients with good upper limb function will want less support in order to maintain their hand function. Some clinical problems may contribute to poor seating. Spasticity of the hamstrings usually pulls on the pelvis causing a posterior tilt, with the patient sitting on the sacrum rather than the ischeal tuberosities. This problem will not just lead to increase risk of pressure sores but can also lead to worsening of a thoracic scoliosis as a compensatory mechanism. Hamstring spasticity should be addressed either medically or surgically. Most patients with severe scoliosis will need foam carved or moulded seats with substantial use of belts and straps to maintain the desired position. Carers should be fully trained to ensure proper transfers and positioning in the seat for the patient. Appropriate seating can improve posture and facilitate care with activities such as feeding but it will not stop progression of the scoliosis.

Orthotic management is very valuable for patients with idiopathic scoliosis as it can correct and stop its progression. Unfortunately, orthoses have a limited role to play in the management of secondary scoliosis, as they are unable to stop its progression. Rigid thoraco lumbar–sacral orthoses may reduce spinal curvature and improve sitting ability while the orthosis is worn. Because the treatment goal is to enable a comfortable and functional sitting posture, over correction may not be indicated. Children with poor levels of sitting ability may demonstrate excessive forward trunk leaning or thoracic kyphosis. Spinal orthoses may prevent forward leaning and improve pulmonary function. Orthotic use for adult patients with secondary scoliosis is neither practical nor effective. Surgical management for secondary scoliosis is also rarely successful.

Further reading

Hart, D. A., McDonald, C. M. (1998). Spinal deformity in progressive neuromuscular disease. *Phys Med Rehabil Clin N Am* **9**, 213–232.
Berven, S., Bradford, D. S. (2002). Neuromuscular scoliosis: causes of deformities and principles for evaluation and management. *Semin Neurol* **22**, 167–178.

Post polio syndrome

A 68-year-old man contracted poliomyelitis when he was nine years old. He was managed initially with a splint, which he used for four years, but afterwards he managed to ambulate independently without using any aids. The patient has had an active life and has been enjoying his retirement for the last three years, being a keen golfer and enjoying walking in the countryside.

Within the last two years, he has noticed increasing fatigue accompanied by a diffuse muscular ache, and his gait has become less steady. He looked on the Internet and suspects that he has post polio syndrome. He is keen to confirm this diagnosis and wants to know if there is anything that can be done to help.

Comments

Despite the World Health Organization's best efforts to eradicate poliomyelitis through a global door-to-door vaccination programme, hundreds of cases are still reported annually, mainly from Nigeria, India and Pakistan where the illness is still endemic. This annual incidence, though unacceptable, could hardly be compared with the hundreds of thousands of patients affected during the peak of the polio epidemic in the early 1950s. Tens of thousands contracted polio in the UK around that time. Fortunately, and within a few years, oral vaccination brought the epidemic to an abrupt end, with almost complete eradication of polio from the Western world by the early 1990s.

Table 6.2. Criteria for the diagnosis of post polio syndrome

---

1. No other medical diagnosis to explain the health problems
2. A confirmed history of paralytic polio
3. Partial neurologic and functional recovery
4. A period of neurological and functional stability of at least 15 years
5. Onset of two or more of the following problems since achieving the period of instability:
   - fatigue
   - muscle and/or joint pain
   - new muscle weakness in muscles previously affected or unaffected
   - new muscle atrophy
   - functional loss
   - cold intolerance

Source: From Halstead and Rossi (1985).

Most of the patients acquiring polio during the peak of its epidemic are in their sixties or early seventies now. Many of them have managed to live a normal and productive life. Therefore, the development of post polio syndrome is usually very distressing.

The prevalence of this syndrome among polio survivors is unknown. Some reports suggested that 25–50% of those infected would develop post polio syndrome at some point. A figure of around 100 000 affected in the UK has been extrapolated from data collected from small populations.

Patients with post polio syndrome usually present with muscle weakness in the already affected muscles or, less commonly in other muscle groups not originally affected by the virus. Muscle atrophy and pain are also common symptoms. Assessment of these symptoms can be difficult as many comorbidities such as arthritis might present in a similar fashion. Generalised fatigue is very common and can become the main reason for disability. It is rare for post polio syndrome to affect the muscles of respiration or swallowing but these impairments are seen in patients with post polio syndrome complicating a severe form of acute polio that left the patient with a life-long significant disability. Exclusion of other causes of the presenting symptoms and signs is an essential diagnostic criterion (Table 6.2).

The prevailing theory explaining the pathology of post polio syndrome is that a degenerative process affects the surviving anterior horn cell neurones. During the stable period following the acute infection, the surviving neurones sprout to provide neuronal supply to the denervated muscles. It is hypothesised that the increased metabolic demands on these surviving neurones makes them more susceptible to early degenerative changes. This hypothesis is consistent with the slow, progressive and unpredictable nature of post polio syndrome.

No pharmacological agent has proven effective in altering the natural history of post polio syndrome or even its common presenting symptoms such as fatigue and muscle weakness. Pain usually responds to standard analgesia. The role of exercise in the management of post polio syndrome used to be controversial as many clinicians had concerns about the potential for exercise and muscular overuse to hasten neural degeneration and muscle fatigue. The prevalent view now is that gentle aerobic exercise is beneficial for the patient as their response to it is identical to the response of normal subjects. Excessive muscle-strengthening exercises, especially using resistance or weights, is usually unsuitable as it has the potential to produce paradoxical weakness of the exercised muscles. However, a trial of a short and gentle strengthening programme early on after diagnosis, with strict monitoring of the patient's muscular function, could be appropriate for selected patients. The exercise prescription should consider the patient's age, lifestyle, comorbidities and the severity of post polio syndrome. In general, the approach to exercise is not dissimilar to the approach and advice given to patients with chronic fatigue syndrome or chronic pain, as most of the patients will have periods of alternating good and bad days, and recommendation of a constant intensity of exercise will not be practical.

Orthotics could be a valuable addition to the patient's management programme. For the suitable patient, it has the potential to reduce pain, increase exercise tolerance and prevent falls and joint deformities. Some patients will have unpleasant memories of heavy and unattractive splints that they used after recovery from the acute attack. Modern orthotics are made from very light material and are more convenient and easier to use.

Assessment of a patient for an orthotic prescription is a complex task as gait abnormalities may be caused by a primary dysfunction of a joint or group of muscles that needs correction or it may be caused by a compensatory mechanism for a primary dysfunction or muscle/joint problem elsewhere. Correction of the compensatory action without addressing the primary cause may lead to worsening of the gait or pain. Elderly patients, in particular, have adapted such compensatory mechanisms for decades, and they may find it difficult to change the pattern of their gait after such a long time.

A simple way to approach the patient clinically is to perform a full clinical examination initially with special emphasis on the ankles, knees and hips for both stability and range of movement. The strength of the main muscle groups affecting these three joints should be evaluated. This should be followed by an assessment of the equality of length between the two legs (by having the patient standing normally and encouraged to take equal pressure on both feet then assessing if there is a difference in level between the anterior superior iliac spines by palpation). Mild differences can easily be corrected using a heel raise, but more significant differences may need heel and sole rises.

Table 6.3. Common clinical impairments, their impact and their orthotic management

Primary abnormality	Biomechanical impact	Clinical impact	Orthotic management
Weak hip abductors	Lean laterally in stance to stabilise the pelvis	Knee valgus deformity; knee pain (*Trendlenberg gait*)	Walking aids
Weak quadriceps	Unable to maintain weight-bearing stability during the stance phase	Knee hyperextension (to lock the knee); knee pain	KAFO; anti-hyperextension knee support (if an isolated problem)
Weak plantar flexors (*calf muscles*)	Unable to control dorsiflexion movement during the mid and late phase of stance (dorsiflexion collapse)	Knee instability during the mid and late stance phase	Rigid dorsiflexion stop AFO; double action ankle joint
Weak dorsiflexors (*tibialis anterior, peronei*)	Inadequate dorsiflexion during the swing phase	Foot drags during swing phase	Passive plantar flexion restraint; active dorsiflexion support[a]
Weak ankle invertors (*tibiali anterior and posterior*)	Medial/lateral ankle instability	Foot collapses on its lateral side (eversion) when weight bearing	Ankle support integrated with an AFO

KAFO, Knee–ankle–foot orthosis; AFO, ankle–foot orthosis;

[a] During mid stance, a rigid AFO will not be able to allow for adequate plantar flexion. This may result in a rapid dorsiflexion, creating a moment around the knee joint leading to knee flexion. A weak quadriceps muscles will be unable to stabilise the knee, with a subsequent worsening of the gait pattern and frequent falls. Because of this complex picture, a KAFO or an AFO with an anti-hyperextension knee support may be needed.

In most of those with post polio syndrome, the abnormalities are complex, with occasional bilateral but asymmetrical distribution. The classic findings are quadriceps weakness with or without weakness of the calf muscles and/or foot dorsiflexors and invertors. These abnormalities are often associated with an unstable hyper extended knee and a valgus foot deformity with a weak plantar and dorsiflexion. Table 6.3 shows the primary problems, their impact and the different strategies to address them.

Reference

Halstead, L. S., Rossi, C. D. (1985). New problems in old polio patients; results of a survey of 539 polio survivors. *Orthopedics* **8**, 845–850.

Further reading

Clark, D. R., Perry, J., Lunsford, T. R. (1986). Case studies: orthotic management of the adult post-polio patient. *Orthot Prosthet* **40**, 43–50.

Perry, J., Clark, D. (1997). Biomechanical abnormalities of postpolio patients and the implication for orthotic management. *Neur Rehabil* **8**, 119–138.

Charcot arthropathy

A 57-year-old man with a long-standing history of type 2 diabetes mellitus was admitted to hospital through the casualty department for the treatment of an ulcer in his right heel. The patient mentioned that he had a minor trauma a few days before when he twisted his right ankle on uneven ground.

The patient was systemically well. Right foot examination showed the discharging ulcer in addition to a distorted foot and ankle with fallen arches. Toenails were abnormally thick and the skin on the foot was hard and showing some callus. Skin over the lower tibia was glistening, with less hair distribution than proximally. The patient had no sensation below the ankle. The patient had good peripheral pulsation on Doppler examination but an ankle brachial pressure index could not be elicited as systolic pressure of his ankle was 240 mm/Hg.

The patient lived alone. Despite being diabetic for a long time, he was not regularly seen by any podiatry or diabetic clinic.

Options for further management were discussed with the patient.

Comments

Charcot arthropathy is a progressive condition characterised by joint dislocations, pathological fractures and debilitating deformities. The disorder results in progressive destruction of bone and soft tissues at weight bearing joints and in its most severe form may cause significant disruption of the bony architecture. The condition can affect any joint; however, it occurs most commonly in the lower extremity at the foot and ankle.

Diabetes mellitus is considered to be the most common cause of Charcot arthropathy, with an incidence of 1–2.5%. However, any condition that causes a sensory or autonomic neuropathy can lead to a Charcot joint. It can occur as a complication of syphilis, chronic alcoholism, leprosy, meningomyelocoele, spinal cord injury, syringomyelia, renal dialysis, or congenital insensitivity to pain.

Two major theories have been proposed to explain the pathophysiology of this condition. The first is the neurotraumatic theory, which suggests that a Charcot joint results from an unperceived trauma or injury to an insensate foot. The sensory neuropathy renders the patient unaware of the osseous destruction that occurs with ambulation. This microtrauma leads to progressive destruction and damage to bone and joints.

The second explanation, the neurovascular theory, suggests that the underlying condition causes development of an autonomic neuropathy. This leads to shunting of blood from the arterioles to venules, reflected by good bouncing pulse on Doppler assessment. This neuropathy causes the extremity to receive increased blood flow and leads to osteopenia through an inbalance in bone destruction and synthesis.

Charcot arthropathy most likely results from a combination of these mechanisms. The autonomic neuropathy leads to abnormal bone formation, and the sensory neuropathy leads to an insensate joint that is susceptible to trauma. In the face of abnormal bone with no ability to protect the joint, the bone gradually becomes fractured and the joint becomes subluxed.

The affected patient can present with either an acute or a chronic arthropathy. Acute Charcot joint almost always presents with signs of inflammation. This is associated with profound unilateral swelling, an increase in local skin temperature, erythema and joint effusion. Instability and loss of joint function may be present. Passive movement of the joint may reveal a 'loose bag of bones.' Despite the general lack of sensation, pain is present in more than 75% of patients. Approximately 40% of patients with acute Charcot arthropathy have concomitant ulceration, thereby complicating the diagnosis and raising concern for osteomyelitis.

Excluding infection is the priority in acute management. The white blood cell count is a non-specific marker for inflammation, and it may be elevated in patients with Charcot arthropathy and no infection. The erythrocyte sedimentation rate is useful but not sensitive enough to confirm the presence of infection. C-reactive protein, an inflammatory marker, is a more reliable test, with a markedly high reading suggesting active infection. It is usually difficult to differentiate between deep soft tissue infection and osteomyelitis. Bone biopsy is the only unequivocal method to establish diagnosis of osteomyelitis. However, CT, MRI or plain radiographs are usually used. The main limitation is the relatively long period between the onset and the appearance of the classic osteomyelitis changes in a radiograph.

The main medical management in the acute condition is to treat the infection with appropriate antibiotics and maintain tight control of blood glucose level, particularly because hyperglycemia can cause non-enzymatic collagen glycosylation, leading to laxity in ligaments and unstable joints.

Protecting the joint is essential. Podiatry input is of great value in the care of skin and toenails to avoid further damage. Patients should not bear weight on an acute Charcot joint. The joint is protected by either a total contact cast or an appropriate orthosis. A Charcot retaining orthotic walker (CROW) is particularly popular as it allows removal of the orthosis for short periods at home for bathing or other activities. Patients with bilateral Charcot arthropathies may need to be confined to a wheelchair to avoid weight bearing on both feet. The period of strict non-weight bearing is usually two to six months.

After healing, continuous protection of the affected foot will be needed. A custom-moulded orthosis would be appropriate for mildly affected Charcot foot. A severe or sublaxed Charcot joint might need a more robust protection with further minimisation of weight bearing. This could be helped by using orthosis such as a patellar tendon bearing AFO.

Some patients with considerable foot instability or recurrent ulcers will require surgical intervention to stabilise and realign the affected foot. Several operations can be useful, such as Achilles tendon lengthening, osteotomies or arthrodesis.

The main indication for amputation of the affected limb is failure to control soft tissue or bone infection. Infection in an insensate diabetic foot may be difficult to combat at the tissue level because of decreased leucocytic activity in the hyperglycemic state. Some patients continue to walk on infected feet, rapidly spreading infected fluids along tissue planes.

The level of amputation required depends mainly on the extent of infection. Transcutaneous oxygen measurement will give reliable information regarding tissue perfusion, which can predict future tissue healing following amputation. Toe, partial foot, Symes and below knee amputations are all options. A few patients need an even higher level, such as above knee amputations. The views of the rehabilitation physicians should be sought prior to amputation as the chosen level and length of the stump will have profound implications in the prosthetic rehabilitation of the affected patient.

The patient will need standard prosthetic management. However, special care should be given to the stump, with regular checks for both the amputated and surviving limbs. A loosely fitted prosthesis should be avoided, especially with a patellar-bearing socket, as this might put excessive pressure on the stump end, which can still show insensate areas, leading to further skin damage. It is occasionally preferred to use total contact sockets with silicon liners to avoid such a problem.

The patient should be encouraged to assess his skin daily, using a mirror or with help of carers. Regular visits to diabetic and podiatry clinics should be arranged.

Further reading

Jeffcoate, W., Lima, J., Nobreqa, L. (2000). The Charcot foot. *Diabet Med* **17**, 253–258.
Elftman, N. W. (2006). Orthotic management of the neuropathic limb. *Phys Med Rehabil Clinic N Am* **17**, 115–157.

7

Ethical and medicolegal controversies

In the last few decades, scientific medicine has evolved in an unimaginable way enabling clinicians to help their patients with either curative measures or with highly effective treatments to relieve their symptoms. However, the same period witnessed the development of new concepts such as human rights and patient's autonomy, which in conjunction with the widespread dissemination of medical information, has empowered patients and put them in a better position to challenge their doctors and question their judgements.

In rehabilitation practice, most decisions are made following a discussion with the patient. Goal setting, in particular, is meaningless if the explicit support of the patient for the goal suggested is not secured. Within such atmosphere, conflicts are not uncommon. The patient may focus on walking as a priority, while the clinicians may feel that independence in self-care is more important as it will help the sitting balance and eventually help the patient achieve his goal of walking. Another patient with detruser sphincter dyssynergia of the bladder may underestimate the risk of renal failure and refuse an inconvenient but safe way to manage his bladder.

Disagreements and conflicts are also common with families and carers, who are often under incredible stress and need significant help to cope with a life-changing event. Occasionally, carers may put pressure on the patient to accept measures with which he/she is not comfortable, leaving the clinicians in a very sensitive position. With the patient's best interest at stake, they must try desperately to balance their role as the patient's advocate with their duty to the family and the importance of respecting the patient's decision.

In a rehabilitation setting, ethical and moral controversies may lack the elements of a successful television/soap medical; nonetheless, the difficulty in dealing with them is no less. Issues such as patient's capacity, discharge destination and end-of-life choices are problems that clinicians have to deal with routinely.

A wandering patient

A 21-year-old man was admitted to the rehabilitation unit three weeks after sustaining a closed head injury while a passenger in a head-on collision. The CT scan was normal and diffuse axonal injury was suggested. On admission to the rehabilitation unit, the patient had no localising neurological signs with the exception of symmetrically brisk tendon reflexes in upper and lower limbs, suggesting recovering tetraparesis.

The patient's mobility improved and within 10 days of admission to the rehabilitation unit, the patient was independently mobile. However, the patient was still confused and disorientated and the clinical psychologist suggested that he still had post-traumatic amnesia.

The patient tended to wander aimlessly in the unit and on several occasions he tried to leave. The staff found it more and more difficult to keep him in and persuade him to stay. A meeting was held with staff, who suggested sedation or at least locking the unit doors. However, nobody seemed sure about the legalities of detaining him.

Comments

Wandering and agitation are common problems following brain injury. Patients are often managed in general medical, surgical or rehabilitation wards, as their problems with agitation and the tendency to wander are usually self-limiting. Traditional interventions to prevent wandering include restraint, drugs, tagging and locked doors.

The detention of those patients who lack the mental capacity to express an informed decision to leave hospital has caused uncertainty and difficulties for clinicians as most of the patients are 'informal', which means that the provisions of the Mental Health Act are not used. The difficulties relate to whether it is lawful to detain and treat informal patients who lack the capacity to express choice.

In emergency situations, the medicolegal framework to manage the wandering patient is straightforward. Common law enables any citizen to intervene if there is an impending danger for the patient himself or others. This situation usually arises if the patient tries to jump out of a window or use stairs while having significant balance problems. The right to interfere verbally or physically is limited to the period of impending danger and ends as the potential risk for the patient or others is removed.

Clarification of the medicolegal framework to manage these patients in the longer term should start with an assessment of the patient's capacity to make treatment choices. Assessment of capacity relates to whether or not a person is able to understand the information relevant to the decision, retain that information, use that information as part of the process of making the decision and finally communicate a decision.

If the patient was deemed to have the capacity to make decisions regarding refusing treatment or leaving the hospital, that decision should not be challenged. If the patient lacks the capacity to make decisions, clinicians in charge should decide if treatment/staying in hospital is necessary as well as being in the patient's best interest. This process should be repeated and further advice sought if difficulties arise. If a patient who does not have capacity to make decisions about treatment tries to leave the ward, measures to ensure the patient's safety that fall short of restraint should be considered. One-to-one supervision, persuasion and distraction are usually effective in diffusing the situation. Clinicians should recognize that restraint could be either physical – including locked doors – or pharmacological.

Despite the lack of robust evidence of their effectiveness, several medications such as antipsychotic and antiepileptic drugs are often prescribed. Antipsychotic drugs in particular have been shown to prolong the period of post-traumatic amnesia and also to have detrimental effects on the cognitive function. Despite the usefulness of such drugs in the management of agitation, their routine use to tackle the problem of wandering is unjustified.

Once the team has decided that restraint is necessary to ensure the safety of the patient or others, the Mental Health Act should be considered. Mental health nurses have the right to detain patients for periods up to 6 hours under Section 5(4) and doctors up to 72 hours under Section 5(2). The aim of these sections is mainly to allow time for assessment of mental state by psychiatrists and use of other sections of the Act if appropriate. Sections 5(4) and 5(2) cannot be renewed; therefore, they cannot be used as a basis for detaining patients for prolonged periods of time.

Environmental and behavioural interventions are the cornerstone of the management of head-injuried patients at this stage. Environmental interventions may include admission to a single quiet room to reduce excessive stimulation. The patient should also have a structured daily routine with timetabled events and rest periods. A consistent approach to these difficulties by staff, families and visitors should also be ensured and Table 7.1 outlines a set of guidelines to support such an approach.

Further reading

Mental Health Act (1983). London: HMSO.

Reidel, D., Shaw, V. (1997). Nursing management of patients with brain injury requiring one to one care. *Rehabil Nurs* **22**, 36–39.

Gaber, T. A. (2006). Medico-legal and ethical aspects in managing wandering patients following traumatic brain injury. *Disabil Rehabil* **28**, 1413–1416.

Table 7.1. Proposed guidelines for management of patients at risk
from wandering

1. Risk assessment should be carried out before mobile head-injuried patients are
   transferred to the rehabilitation unit. If confusion and wandering may be a
   problem, adequate staffing should be arranged to allow one-to-one supervision and
   structured daily activities
2. If the patient attempts to leave the unit, persuasion/distraction should be tried
3. The patient's family should be informed that if the patient is determined to leave
   the unit the intention is either to let him go or to invoke the Mental Health Act
   under a relevant section. The wishes of the family should be documented
   and considered
4. If the patient is determined to leave the unit, the nurse in charge jointly with
   the team should decide either to let the patient go, and inform the family,
   police and the social worker, or to contact the doctor to consider invoking
   Section 5(2) and to allow time to contact the mental health team for an assessment
   for other sections of the Act. The decision should be based on:
   • earlier discussions with the family/team
   • situation in the ward and the risk of trying to restrain the patient versus the
     potential risk for the patient if left to go
5. A pathway should be negotiated with the local mental health team and three
   important issues should be clarified
   • Contact number/person 24 hours a day
   • Time scale for assessment under the Mental Health Act
   • Whether the patient will stay in the rehabilitation ward or transfer to a mental
     health facility

Source: From Gaber, T. (2006). *Disabil Rehabil* **28**, 1413–1416, with permission (www.
informaworld.com).

Rehabilitation of the patient from an ethnic minority

A 72-year-old Asian woman was admitted to the rehabilitation unit following a head injury after a fall. The patient used to be independent and in
normal health before the fall. She spoke very little English; however, the
rehabilitation unit staff managed to work with her to improve her mobility
and independence. The patient's family noticed some cognitive impairment and reported this to the staff. It was difficult to formally assess her
cognitive function owing to the language difficulties. Despite several
family meetings, the patient and her family did not seem happy with the
progression of the rehabilitation programme.

Comments

The process of rehabilitation requires patients to be actively engaged and to adopt a higher level of interaction with healthcare professionals than in other medical settings. Current models of rehabilitation are dictated by Western values, expectations, priorities and health beliefs, which may have limited relevance to people from ethnic minority communities. In the developed world, individual autonomy and independence are values that are cherished by all patients, who will naturally subscribe to these as the main objectives of a successful rehabilitation programme.

Rehabilitation staff may try to foster such perceived majority attitudes in all patients regardless of their ethnic background. Asian and Middle Eastern ethnic groups, in particular, have well-established social structures and family values that evolved to ensure the welfare of the elderly and vulnerable in a potentially hostile, tribal social structure where the state rarely played any significant role in providing health or financial support for elderly or disabled people . At the heart of these values is the duty of the family to care for elderly people. Members of the family ignoring such duties will be a source of disgrace and shame in a community where family honour is a prime concern.

In a rehabilitation setting, family members will naturally be keen for their relative to improve physically and cognitively. Occasionally, they may struggle to grasp the rational of going to great lengths to ensure independence in a particular activity of daily living as they feel that it would be much easier for them to help their relative to perform such a task. Elderly patients, in particular, will consider it the duty of their sons and daughters to provide all essential care for them and might find it absurd that they should struggle to do a particular activity while their family is around.

These different ways of looking at the role of the family are not the only significant challenge facing the rehabilitation professionals. Patients from ethnic minorities can be more susceptible to certain illnesses, with, for example, a higher incidence of diabetes mellitus. Those comorbidities may complicate the rehabilitation process. Patients from ethnic minorities are not only more likely to have mental health problems such as anxiety and depression but they may also be more reluctant to admit it and be open about their feelings. Therefore, they can present with different psychosomatic symptoms, which, in conjunction with the language barrier, can make it extremely difficult to evaluate the patient objectively.

The impact of these challenges could be minimised if the rehabilitation team were adequately equipped to serve this group of patients. It would be sensible if all members of the rehabilitation team had formal training in cultural awareness, especially in teams serving a population with a significant ethnic mix. Assessment of the patient should highlight any potential issues that may have an impact on the rehabilitation process, such as language barriers, patients' beliefs about illnesses, and social situations. Any problem should be tackled appropriately. While language barriers can be addressed with an interpreter service, it is also important that staff should try to develop a mechanism to deal with patients' needs around the clock. Language barriers have significant impact in patients with cognitive or behavioural impairments as it will be almost impossible to use any standardised psychometric tests. A more informal approach to cognitive rehabilitation would be appropriate in most cases.

All rehabilitation goals should be discussed with the patient and the family, with an explanation of the rationale of using specific methods; for example, a particular physiotherapy programme will not necessarily strengthen muscles or improve mobility but it may tackle a high muscle tone or maintain the range of movement of joints. The goals should be explicit and the views of the patient should always be considered; for example, a Muslim patient may prefer washing in the morning to be replaced by washing for prayer at an earlier time.

Patients from ethnic minorities may suffer from social isolation, especially if they are recently arrived immigrants. Conversely, some patients will have a large number of relatives in the locality. Both scenarios carry the potential for a complicated discharge. The socially isolated patient may need more support resources in the community as he/she may lack some of the social skills and *know-how* that the average patient has. Patients with large families often refuse care provided by agencies other than their immediate family members as they consider this to be the family's duty. This approach may lead to considerable stress and burden on a young family, especially the daughter-in-law as she is traditionally the person responsible for the day-to-day care of the elderly father or mother. Stress in the carers should be assessed as the patient is followed up.

Further reading

Niemeiere, J. P., Burnett, D. M., Whitaker, D. A. (2003). Cultural competence in multidisciplinary rehabilitation setting: are we falling short of meeting needs? *Arch Phys Med Rehabil* **84**, 1240–1245.

Eshiett, M. U., Parry, E. H. (2003). Migrants and health: a cultural dilemma. *Clin Med* **3**, 229–231.

Service provision for chronic fatigue syndrome

Funding for a specialist service for patients with chronic fatigue syndrome (CFS) was approved locally thanks mainly to intensive lobbying by the local patients' support group. Several models of service provision were suggested. There was general disagreement between the clinical team responsible for the service and the patients' support group regarding the staffing and interventions provided by the service.

Comments

Despite the overwhelming evidence that CFS is at least partly caused by a genuine immunological dysfunction, many clinicians feel that it is a purely psychological illness and a few of them do not even believe that it exists at all. As the diagnosis of CFS is clinical (Table 7.2) and mainly made by exclusion (Table 7.3) with no diagnostic test, it is not unusual to have patients diagnosed months or years after the onset. When the diagnosis is made, the patients may face an indifferent and occasionally hostile attitude from their clinicians. Patients are usually offered physiotherapy, graded exercise being the main recommendation. Despite its proven positive effect in CFS, graded exercise can cause a considerable deterioration if the patient is in a relapse or if it is supervised by a therapist with no experience in treating the condition. A patient may suffer for years before the diagnosis is made, being dismissed

Table 7.2. Fukuda criteria for the diagnosis of chronic fatigue syndrome

	Symptoms
1. Absolute symptom	Fatigue that is • Medically unexplained • Of new onset • Of at least 6 months' duration • Not the result of increased exertion • Not substantially relieved by rest • Causing a substantial reduction of previous vocational, educational, social or personal levels of activities
2. Plus four or more of a second group of symptoms	Self-reporting symptoms of loss of short-term memory and concentration Sore throat Tender cervical or axillary glands Muscle pain Headaches of new type or severity Unrefreshing sleep Post-exertional malaise lasting for at least 24 hours Multijoint pain without swelling or redness

Source: From Fukuda *et al.* (1994).

Table 7.3. Conditions that exclude the diagnosis of chronic fatigue syndrome

Established medical disorder that is known to cause chronic fatigue
Major depressive illness with or without psychosis
Any medication which cause fatigue as a side effect
Eating disorders
Alcohol or substance abuse

by doctors and told that 'it is all in the mind' then exposed to an intervention that makes him/her feels significantly worse.

Considering this potential sequence of events, it is not surprising that many patients take a defensive and sceptical attitude towards the medical establishment. Most patients reject the notion that the illness is mainly psychological outright and go on a quest to find a cure somewhere else. Patients usually gather in well-organised support groups, which provide valuable support and source of information on one hand but occasionally act as a vehicle to promote unproven and occasionally bizarre theories about the origins of the disease, and treatment methods that are not based on any credible evidence.

Support groups for CFS are very organised and effective in lobbying for resources and recognition. In 1998, The UK Chief Medical Officer commissioned a working group to advice him about the most effective methods to manage CFS. The committee membership included professionals and patients' representatives. The work of the group was hindered by several resignations because of the divisions between professionals endorsing a biopsychosocial approach to CFS and patients' representatives insisting on adopting a biomedical method in dealing with sufferers.

The main controversy is that the only two interventions proven to improve the symptoms of CFS and the patient's function are graded exercise and cognitive–behaviour therapy. These two interventions are generally unpopular with patients. No medical intervention has proved effective in CFS. So, what should a CFS specialised service provide to its users?

Extensive consultations with user groups are extremely important. Provision of a 'one size fits all' model with the proven interventions prescribed to all patients is inappropriate. A rehabilitation model of practice with assessment, goal setting, intervention then reviewing the goals will provide a suitable approach to such a heterogeneous group of patients, who differ markedly in the severity of illness, expectations and approach to therapy. Symptom relief and reduction of disability and handicap are traditionally the main outcomes aimed for by a standard rehabilitation programme.

Staffing of the team may vary from the standard rehabilitation services model. Many therapists found that integration of cognitive–behavioural therapy methods during the consultations or therapy sessions might be more appropriate than providing such therapy as a stand-alone session. Graded activities could replace graded exercise as a way to improve fitness level and the patient's function. This should subsequently lead to expanding the patient's social and vocational roles.

The team members should have some flexibility in their approach to their professional roles. Adequate training should be provided to all staff not only regarding CFS but also in the basics of cognitive–behavioural therapy. Medical input for support, explanation and symptom control should be available to selected patients.

Up to 20% of patients with CFS suffer from a severe and debilitating form of the disease and many of them are bed bound. A CFS service must have protocols and plans to deal with such a difficult and complex group of patients. Home visits are usually needed; however, the chances of significant improvement with just community input alone are very limited. There are a few inpatient facilities in the UK that specialise in severe CFS, adopting usually a model of an intensive inpatient rehabilitation programme. The published research appraising such an approach is very limited. The prevailing impression is that inpatient rehabilitation programmes are often successful, leading to significant improvement in the patients' functional abilities in the short term. The long-term outcome is less certain.

Children suffering with CFS will have different needs, as continuing schooling and education is one of the most important management goals. It is very difficult for a CFS adult service team to possess the necessary skills that enable them to deal with affected children with their unique problems and needs. The team members of the children's service should ideally have a paediatric background in either nursing or therapy. Paediatricians or child and adolescent psychiatrists can provide valuable medical or mental health input.

Reference

Fukuda, K., Strauss, S. E., Hickie, I. B., *et al.* (1994). Chronic fatigue syndrome: a comprehensive approach to its definition and management. *Ann Intern Med* **121**, 953–959.

Further reading

Cox, D. L. (1998). The management of chronic fatigue syndrome: development and evaluation of a dedicated service. *Br J Ther Rehabil* **5**, 205–209.

Sharpe, M. (2002). The report of the Chief Medical Officer's CFS/ME working group: what does it say and will it help? *Clin Med* **2**, 427–429.

8

Chronic pain

Pain is a common problem in neurologically impaired patients. Establishing the cause of pain should not be the only objective of clinical assessment. The severity of pain and its impact on the patient's life are important as they present the clinician with the best tools to monitor the effects of the management plan. Rating the severity of pain using a scale of 1 to 10 is a simple severity measurement tool. Questions regarding sleep pattern or mood can provide a basic indication of the influence pain is having on the patient's life and will enable the clinician to integrate different strategies into the standard medical management to try to maintain the patient's activities. Sleep is very important, and following a good sleep hygiene can in itself improve the overall picture.

Chronic pain is strongly associated with the patient's mood and beliefs. Some services will have access to cognitive–behavioural therapy, which will be a valuable component of the overall management plan. For immobile patients, postural abnormalities often accentuate pain, especially spinal and lower limb pain. Physiotherapy assessment may be needed to exclude such problems in selected patients.

Establishing the prognosis is an important component of the clinical assessment. Conditions such as painful spasms or restless leg syndrome can be adequately controlled in many patients. Patients with neuropathic pain or spinal pain respond less favourably to treatment, and a discussion with the patient before commencement of therapy should focus on discussing the patient's expectations and encouraging a realistic view of what can be achieved. An ongoing litigation is a very poor prognostic factor for patients with chronic pain.

Central pain syndrome

A 64-year-old woman presented to the rehabilitation clinic three months after having a left hemisphere stroke that left her with dense right hemiplegia and global aphasia. The patient's family reported that the patient seemed to have pain and discomfort most of the time. The patient's physiotherapist said that the patient was unable to tolerate even touching the affected arm, with hypersensitivity of the skin on that side. Clinical examination was very difficult because of her communication impairment, but the patient seemed to be in extreme discomfort when trying to touch or move her right arm.

Comments

The term central pain syndrome refers to the pain phenomenon occurring secondary to a spinothalamic tract lesion. The pathology can affect the thalamus directly or any of its connections with either the cortical sensory centres or the peripheral connections to the spinal cord. Stroke is one of the commonest causes of central pain with 8% of stroke sufferers developing it. Patients with post-stroke sensory impairment are more vulnerable to central pain syndrome, with an incidence of up to 20% in this group. Patients presenting with a post-stroke central pain usually have multiple brain lesions showing in their scans, with supratentorial lesions generally producing pain in the extremities and infratentorial lesions leading to facial pain.

The pain usually starts immediately after the stroke but around half of the patients will develop the syndrome more than a month after the onset of their stroke. The pain character varies significantly between patients, with burning, aching, pins and needles, or crushing or lacerating characters to the pain usually described. Despite such variable presentations, severity of pain is almost universally very intense, with **allodynia** reported in more than 70% of patients. In those with allodynia, normal tactile or cold sensations will provoke intense unpleasant pain. Movement of the affected limb can also provoke the same response, and this will subsequently impact on the patient's rehabilitation as any residual motor function will be very difficult to utilise in a functional way and even passive movement to maintain the range of movement of joints can be difficult.

Post-stroke central pain syndrome was first described more than 100 years ago. However, drug trials to improve pain control are rare, and amitriptyline and lamotrigine are the only medications proven to improve pain control in randomised trials. In common with other neuropathic pain syndromes, simple analgesia, NSAIDs and opiate derivatives are of limited value, and most patients report no effect on the pain even when using strong opiates. Tricyclic antidepressants and antiepileptic drugs are the traditional medications used in management. The mode of action of tricyclic antidepressants in neuropathic pain is poorly understood, with some authors suggesting that the analgesic action is mainly a by-product of the improvement in mood and the mildly sedative effect. The mode of action of the antiepileptic drugs, by comparison, is relatively easy to predict as their main mode of action, whether it is sodium channel blockade or GABA transmitter agonism, should eventually lead to inhibition of neuronal excitation and subsequent reduction in the firing of the pain-producing neurones. This favourable mode of action may come with less-welcomed side effects, such as sedation or mental slowness, which all patients should be warned of as potential problems. Many of these side effects ease off as the dose is built up, and patients should be encouraged to try to persevere with mild side effects in the hope that they will improve with time.

As mentioned above, lamotrigine is the only antiepileptic proven to help post-stroke central pain. This is definitely in keeping with the author's experience. Lamotrigine is not licensed for pain in the UK. The literature suggests a dose of 200 mg daily as the usual maintenance dose. A patient not responding to such a dosage will probably not respond to a higher dose. If the patient fails to respond to or tolerate lamotrigine, other antiepileptic drugs such as gabapentin or carbamazepine could be tried.

In patients with spinal injuries or multiple sclerosis, central pain is common, with 66% of patients with multiple sclerosis reporting pain and 25% reporting severe pain that significantly affects their quality of life. In both groups of patients, pain can result from different pathologies and mechanisms. Therefore, careful clinical assessment is mandatory to establish the exact cause, as problems such as painful muscular spasms and musculoskeletal pain are common and their management differs from that for central pain.

In multiple sclerosis, neuropathic pain can present as trigeminal neuralgia, radicular pain or a spinothalamic (central) pain. Clinicians should remember that up to 5% of these patients could have peripheral neuropathy as a part of their neurological presentation, with the peripheral neuropathy occasionally presenting with a classic painful peripheral neuropathic syndrome.

Spinothalamic pain associated with either spinal injury or multiple sclerosis is usually severe and resistant to treatment. Again, tricyclic antidepressants and antiepileptic drugs are the usual drug classes used. There is no strong evidence to suggest the superiority of one drug above another. A reasonable approach to management is to start with the drugs with the least side effects, such as gabapentin or lamotrigine, moving on to more potent antiepileptic drugs such as sodium valproate if necessary. For resistant pain, I usually try topiramate, which is very potent but can be difficult to tolerate. Starting with a small dose and building it up very slowly can increase the chances of a successful titration and eventually a satisfactory control of the pain. In central pain secondary to spinal injury or multiple sclerosis, strong slow-release opiate derivatives can be a useful add-on therapy.

One of the problems commonly seen with patients with multiple sclerosis is fatigue. Many patients fail to tolerate tricyclic antidepressants or antiepileptic drugs because of the deterioration of their fatigue or the increased sedation. The management plan will always be a trade off between the pain relief and the worsening of fatigue or other side effects.

Synthetic canabinoid is available for some forms of pain in those with multiple sclerosis. As well as helping with pain, it can also reduce the frequency and severity of spasms and fatigue. The exact role it can play in the management of central pain is still controversial.

For intractable pain not responding to medical management, neurosurgical advice should always be sought. Procedures such as spinal cord stimulation and deep brain stimulation have been performed for years with variable results. More recently motor cortex stimulation has become the preferred procedure for the management of central pain. The procedure can improve the pain in 50–75% of those affected. The main clinical challenge is the selection of patients who possess the best chance of responding to these neurostimulation techniques.

Further reading

Andersen, G., Vestergaard, K., Ingeman-Nielsen, M., et al. (1995). Incidence of central post-stroke pain. *Pain* **61**, 187–193.

Nguyen, J. P., Lefaucher, J. P., Le-Guerinel, C., et al. (2000). Motor cortex stimulation in the treatment of central and neuropathic pain. *Arch Med Res* **31**, 263–265.

Solaro, C. (2006). Epidemiology and treatment of pain in multiple sclerosis. *Neurol Sci* **27** (Suppl. 4), s291–s293.

Complex regional pain syndrome

A 22-year-old man presented with persistent pain and swelling affecting the left ankle two months after he had an ankle sprain. Clinically, the patient avoided weight bearing on the affected ankle. The whole left foot was swollen, with significant allodynia and mild sensory changes. The left foot colour, temperature and hair distribution were similar to the right foot. The patient reported noticing occasional changes in the affected foot's temperature and sweating in relation to the rest of the body.

Comments

The term complex regional pain syndrome (CRPS) was coined in the mid-1990s to describe a spectrum of pain syndromes that have chronic pain, disability and autonomic dysfunction as their cardinal manifestations. The term is gradually replacing a myriad of names that used to describe the illness such as reflex sympathetic dystrophy, causalgia, Sudeck syndrome and shoulder–hand syndrome. Reflex sympathetic dystrophy (RSD) is a

Table 8.1. Definition of complex regional pain syndrome from the International Association for the Study of Pain

A variety of painful conditions that usually:

- follow injury
- occur regionally
- have a distal predominance of abnormal findings
- exceed in both magnitude and duration the expected course of the inciting event
- result in marked impairment of motor function
- are associated with oedema, abnormal skin blood flow, or vasomotor activity in the region of the pain at some time during the course of the illness

From Bruehl *et al.* (1999).

term recognised by many patients and clinicians; therefore, many authors prefer to use RSD/CRPS as a more inclusive name. The condition can occur at any age and is not uncommon in children. The literature suggests an incidence of 1–2 % of CRPS after bony fractures and 2–5 % after peripheral nerve injuries.

There are two types of CRPS. Type 1 follows an injury that can vary in severity, and occasionally it is so mild that the patient fails to even remember it. The injury usually leads to immobilisation. In Type 2, an injury will lead to well-recognised nerve damage. In both types, the injury will be followed by a disproportional pain in conjunction with a multitude of symptoms such as allodynia (painful response to normally non-noxious stimulus) or hyperalgesia (heightened response to a painful stimulus). The pain syndrome is often associated with symptoms and signs of vasomotor dysfunction, such as discolouration, increase or decrease in sweating, hair loss or oedema (Table 8.1).

Early diagnosis of CRPS is extremely important as early intervention with mobilisation, adequate pain relief and psychological support can improve the prognosis significantly. A long-standing CRPS has a very poor prognosis, and treatment is usually very difficult at this stage. However, resolution of the symptoms can occur at any stage.

One factor that affects early diagnosis of the condition is that the clinical vasomotor signs are intermittent, and their absence at one consultation does not necessarily exclude their presence. The signs can also vary in severity with time. Allodynia is an important clinical sign, which should alert the examining clinician to the possibility of CRPS. A long list of conditions can present in a similar fashion and the differential diagnoses should be considered in all patients (Table 8.2). Several investigations can aid the clinical diagnosis such as plain radiograph, which may show evidence of localised osteopenia.

Table 8.2. Differential diagnosis of complex regional pain syndrome

Fractures
Other causes of neuropathy
Cellulitis
Septic arthritis
Lyme disease
Neurosarcoidosis
Polycythaemia vera
Peripheral nerve neuroma
Raynaud's disease

Thermography and three-phase bone scintigraphy can show specific changes and MRI can also aid the diagnosis by excluding other pathologies such as stress fractures.

Motor complications are common in severe cases and they can vary from ignoring the use of the affected limb, in a way that is not dissimilar to the behaviour seen in cognitive neglect phenomenon, to severe weakness and dystonia. Another serious complication is migration of the condition to other parts of the body, affecting usually other extremities and less commonly central areas like the neck and trunk.

Physiotherapy and occupational therapy in conjunction with psychological support are the cornerstones of management. The rehabilitation effort could be underestimated by the patient in quest of a pharmacological cure. The rehabilitation programme will depend on the severity of the condition, but a standard approach will be to start with desensitisation by light touch and then moving to passive and active mobilisation to maintain the range of movement. Strengthening exercises including weight bearing can start under the cover of adequate analgesia. Several associated conditions could be helped with therapy, such as oedema or temperature disturbances. Methods such a functional electrical stimulation are commonly used, but the evidence for their effectiveness is lacking. The standard rehabilitation programme should address the social and vocational issues as well.

When using analgesia, the patient should remain aware that the objective of the medications is to encourage continued movement of the limb. The effects of the medication prescribed should be evaluated as objectively as possible. Antidepressants and antiepileptic drugs remain the most popular drugs used. Other medications such as bisphosphonates have been tried, with pamidronate showing promising results especially in CRPS affecting the ankle.

Invasive techniques such as sympathetic block are popular. Most clinicians start with an intravenous sympathetic block. If successful, they offer the patient a destructive sympathetic ganglion block. Evaluation of such a technique is difficult because of the heterogeneity of the CRPS presentation. Again, the patient should accept that the syndrome is more than pain and should use any period of pain relief to try to improve the affected limb function. Spinal dorsal root stimulator is another invasive technique that can be offered to selected patients.

Reference

Bruehl, S., Harden, R. N., Galer, B. S., *et al.* (1999). External validation of IASP diagnostic criteria for complex regional pain syndrome and proposed research diagnostic criteria. Internation Association for the Study of Pain. *Pain* **81**, 147–154.

Further reading

Marshall, A. T., Crisp, A. J. (2000). Reflex sympathetic dystrophy. *Rheumatology* **39**, 692–695.

Burton, A. W., Hassenbusch, S. J., Warneke, C., *et al.* (2004). Complex regional pain syndrome: a survey of current practices. *Pain Pract* **4**, 74–83.

Stanton-Hicks, M., Baron, R., Boas, R. (1998). Complex regional pain syndrome: guidelines for therapy. *Clin J Pain* **14**, 155–166.

Shoulder pain following stroke

A 64-year-old man was admitted to hospital following collapse at home. The patient had left-sided weakness. A CT scan showed right parietal and temporal lobe infarction.

During the patient's rehabilitation, one of the main problems was his left upper limb, which showed sensory impairment, complete flaccid paralysis and shoulder pain. Clinically, the left shoulder showed a distance of 2 cm between the acromion and the head of the humerus, indicating shoulder subluxation.

Comments

Loss of arm function is a common and devastating outcome of stroke. About three quarters of the patients initially show a motor deficit in the upper limb and recovery is generally poor. Rehabilitation of the upper limb is difficult, with only 5% of stroke survivors who have complete paralysis regaining functional use of their impaired arm and hand. Shoulder pain is also a common problem following stroke and can delay rehabilitation and functional recuperation as the painful joint may mask any improvement of motor function. Shoulder pain can affect up to 70% of patients and often appears in the first few days.

The vulnerability of the shoulder is easily appreciated once its anatomical structure is considered. Three bones, humerus, clavicle and scapula, together with more than 30 muscles, constitute and control the movements of this extremely mobile joint. The wide range of movement of the shoulder helps the subject to locate his/her, hand in space enabling a wide range of hand functional tasks to be achieved.

The following processes have all been postulated as potential causes of a painful hemiplegic shoulder: gleno humeral subluxation, spasticity of shoulder muscles, impingement, soft tissue trauma, rotator cuff tears, glenohumeral capsulitis, biceps tendonitis and shoulder–hand syndrome. Early intervention is essential to prevent the development of shoulder joint contracture.

A careful assessment of the shoulder can often indicate the pathology, such as muscle spasticity or adhesive capsulitis, which may be amenable to a specific intervention. Assessment should always start with careful observation and inspection of both the normal and the affected shoulders, observing any abnormal posture or muscle wasting. A fingerbreadth palpable gap between the acromion and the humeral head would suggest joint subluxation. In a paralysed shoulder, examination of the active range of movement of the shoulder may be impossible. The passive range should be determined in both shoulders. The specific movements precipitating pain should be documented. A painless restricted range of movement suggests adhesive capsulitis as the primary pathology.

The impingement syndrome is a mechanical condition affecting the rotator cuff muscles and commonly results in tendonitis, bursitis or rotator cuff tear. The rotator cuff muscles are the group of muscles that originate from the scapula and insert in the head of humerus, forming a cuff (Table 8.3). The main function of these muscles is to stabilise the shoulder. The tendons of the rotator cuff muscles are very vulnerable to inflammation and tears and are implicated in many of the shoulder pain syndromes.

Treatment for hemiplegic shoulder pain aims at dealing with the patient's pain in the early and often flaccid stage when the shoulder is prone to inferior subluxation and traction on the glenohumeral capsule, which may lead to damage of the brachial plexus or soft tissues. Different strategies are often implemented in rehabilitation of the patient in order to achieve the best outcome. The ideal management of hemiplegic stroke pain is to prevent it happening in the first place. Support for the limb is important during the early stages and there are different ways of achieving this. Adequate positioning of the upper limb reduces the tension placed on the anatomical structures of the shoulder joint and the muscles and nerves surrounding it.

Table 8.3. Rotator cuff muscles

Name	Origin	Insertion	Function
Supraspinatus	Medial two thirds of the supraspinous fossa	Upper facet of the humerus	Initiates abduction at the shoulder (first 20 degrees); holds head of humerus firmly against glenoid fossa to prevent upward shearing of the humeral head when deltoid takes over abduction phase (20 degrees plus)
Subscapularis	Medial two thirds of the subscapular fossa and from tendinous septa	Lesser tubercle of the humerus	Strong medial rotator of the shoulder; may also assist in adduction of the arm
Infraspinatus	Medial two thirds of the infraspinous fossa of the scapula	Middle facet of the greater tubercle of the humerus	Lateral rotator of the arm
Teres minor	Two heads: upper two thirds of the lateral border of the scapula and the fascia between it	Lowest facet on the greater tubercle of the humerus	Lateral rotator When the arm is abducted, it laterally rotates and adducts

The multidisciplinary team, the patient and carers must also be informed on how to position the paralysed arm in order to avoid injuries to the shoulder. Slings and supports can be used in order to provide additional support for the flaccid upper limb. However, the upper limb must be positioned where it is not at potential risk of further damage: if support is not reducing the degree of subluxation or tension on the joint then it is at risk of damage. Strapping has been advocated during the early phase, but skin damage through the taping is a potential risk; hence frequent monitoring of the taping and the patient's sensory awareness of the upper limb is essential when applying the tape.

Stimulation of the upper limb with transcutaneous electrical nerve stimulation or functional electrical stimulation can be used to elicit a muscle contraction and also for pain relief. The latter has demonstrated beneficial effect on subluxation and shoulder pain, range of motion and arm function in a few studies, but one main potential disadvantage of these methods of stimulation is the potential for deterioration after withdrawal of the external stimulus.

Later on in the rehabilitation of the patient, muscle spasticity may occur and limit the range of movement. Relieving spasticity through specific handling/mobilisation and drug treatment should be considered as it may lead to significant improvement of the shoulder pain and range of movement.

Further reading

Bender, L., McKenna, K. (2001). Hemiplegic shoulder pain: defining the problem and its management. *Disabil Rehabil* **23**, 698–705.

Turner-Stokes, L., Jackson, D. (2002). Shoulder pain after stroke: a review of evidence base to inform the development of an integrated care pathway. *Clin Rehabil* **16**, 276–298.

Walsh, K. (2001). Management of shoulder pain in patients with stroke. *Postgrad Med J* **77**, 645–649.

9

Medically unexplained disorders

The medical model of diagnosis and management depends on taking a clinical history, examining the patient and then requesting appropriate investigations. Ideally, this will lead to a diagnosis and formulation of a management plan. Considering this model, it is easy to appreciate the frustration of the treating clinicians when dealing with patients with medically unexplained disorders, as the history is usually non-specific, clinical examination and investigations show no abnormality and the pathology and diagnosis are duly unclear.

Medically unexplained disorders will fit more comfortably with the rehabilitation model of dealing with illness. A focus on disability and handicap is the cornerstone of rehabilitation practice. The nature or severity of the disability and handicap are not necessarily a direct consequence of the pathology or impairment. An epileptic may have pathology but no impairment or disability. However, the impact of the epilepsy on the patient's social or vocational activities may be substantial. A patient with chronic back pain may have no pathology, but the impairment and disability will be significant.

This different way of thinking puts the rehabilitation specialists in a better position when dealing with patients suffering from a medically unexplained disorder. Rehabilitation services are also used routinely to explore social, psychological and vocational issues. These factors are usually the main targets for intervention in such patients.

Conversion syndrome

A 22-year-old woman developed a sudden right arm paralysis. The patient had no risk factors for cerebrovascular disease and the neurological examination showed weakness of the right arm, which was not associated with any pyramidal or peripheral nerve signs. An MRI of the brain and cervical spine, nerve conduction studies and electromyography (EMG) were all normal. The diagnosis of conversion syndrome was suggested.

Comments

Conversion syndrome is a spectrum of disorders that spread along a continuum with the patient's *volition* being the major factor to determine her/his position in that continuum. Patients with complete absence of volition or ability to control the symptoms usually present with the conversion syndrome as an isolated impairment and often have a surprisingly normal mental health profile and social circumstances. At the other end of the spectrum are patients with significant mental health issues and complex social problems including childhood traumas (e.g. abuse). These patients can usually control their symptoms but the impulsivity and the need to produce the symptoms is overwhelming, and the patient's voluntary control is limited. This group of patients should not be confused with malingerers or patients with Munchausen's syndrome, who have almost complete insight and control of their symptoms.

Initial assessment of the patient should aim at determining the patient's position in this continuum, as this position will determine the prognosis and the approach to management. Patients with complex mental health and social issues could paradoxically be easier to manage and more responsive to intervention, as many of these precipitating problems are responsive to appropriate interventions. By comparision, patients presenting with conversion syndrome as an isolated impairment are more difficult to manage.

Explaining the diagnosis is a sensitive task and can make or break the doctor–patient relationship. The patient should be told the diagnosis in an unambiguous manner. Terms like hysterical or 'in the mind' should be avoided. Calling the symptoms functional is usually helpful and acceptable to the patient. I personally use the hardware/software analogy when explaining the symptoms to the patients, telling them that the hardware in their body (e.g. brain, nerves and muscles) are normal but the problem is with the software, meaning that the way these organs are working is affected and leading to the impairment and disability. Most patients find this analogy reassuring and also helpful in setting the stage to the approach taken to manage the disability. Patients with pseudo-seizures usually appreciate the analogy with a 'pressure cooker', like steam, with stress having to express itself in one way or another. A patient accepting this explanation may accept a psychosocial approach to the management of the seizures instead of insisting on pursuing further investigations to establish the cause of his symptoms.

Ideally, a multidisciplinary team should manage the patient, as different facets and dimensions of the disability should be managed simultaneously.

Table 9.1. Cognitive–behavioural therapy

Intervention	Components
Cognitive	Accept that symptoms are genuine but explain that improvement is possible by implementation of a rational treatment strategy
	Challenge negative beliefs regarding the origin of the symptoms (fear of having multiple sclerosis is very common) and that particular activities such as exercise might worsen the symptoms
	Challenge 'catastrophisation cognition' in which the patient may get warning signs of dissociation that will be interpreted as the onset of a serious symptom such as pseudo-seizures
	Tackle the obvious obstacles to recovery such as secondary gain, social or vocational situations
Behavioural	Identify specific behaviours that might be linked with worsening of symptoms
	Graded exposure to feared situations
	Use of relaxation strategies to reduce anxiety symptoms
	Distraction and refocusing techniques to divert attention away from symptoms

A single team managing the patient should also help to provide a consistent explanation of the symptoms and approach to management. Medically, the patient should be offered frequent appointments in the initial stage, either by the GP or a specialist if appropriate. These visits should be used to reassure the patient that the symptoms are taken seriously, to tackle any developing symptoms and to prevent any further inappropriate referrals or investigations. Mental health problems should be managed aggressively. There is evidence that antidepressants can often be beneficial even if the patient is not clinically depressed. Some patients decline antidepressants use, either because of the stigma of mental illness or because of fear of tolerance or addiction. The rationale of using antidepressants should be explained to the patient as an intervention worth exploring.

A specialist psychological assessment is mandatory to identify the psychological predisposing, precipitating or perpetuating factors and to determine how the patient's current cognitive, behavioural and emotional factors exacerbate the somatic symptoms. This assessment should assist with the formulation of the patient's management plan, which usually include cognitive–behavioural therapy (Table 9.1), problem-solving therapy and a family systemic therapy. The implementation of this plan should ideally be carried out by all the members of the team and be integrated in the patient's therapy sessions. Selected patients will need a one-to-one psychological intervention.

Many dilemmas face the clinicians working with a patient with conversion syndrome. The need for equipment or mobility aids could be considered, on the one hand, as enforcing the patient's disability behaviour. On the other hand, such equipment and aids could facilitate the patient's integration with society and play a major role in reducing the handicap. The team should not have rigid rules and policies regarding the provision of such aids, as every patient will be different and careful assessment of the patient's needs should be weighed against the risks of reinforcing the disability.

Another contentious issue is the secondary gain, whether it is financial or emotional/social. Sometimes such gains are substantial, with significant financial gain from benefits or compensation and/or enhancement of the patient's ability to maintain a dependent relationship with family or partner. The secondary gains should be considered in the initial assessment, as high secondary gains are a very poor prognostic factor. Such sensitive issues may be very difficult to discuss with the patient. Again, a decision to tackle this issue or not should be taken on an individual basis.

Further reading

Solyom, C., Solyom, L. A. (1990). Treatment program for functional paraplegia/Munchausen syndrome. *J Behav Ther Exp Psychiatry* **21**, 225–230.

Speed, J. (1996). Behavioral management of conversion disorder: retrospective study. *Arch Phys Med Rehabil* **77**, 147–154.

Stone, J., Carson, A., Sharp, M. (2005). Functional symptoms in neurology: management. *J Neurol Neurosurg Psychiatry* **76**, 13–21.

Somatisation in multiple sclerosis

A 42-year-old woman attended the neurology clinic and asked for steroid therapy as she felt that her multiple sclerosis was relapsing. The patient had been diagnosed with mutiple sclerosis six years previous after a single attack of demyelination, which left her with mild lower limb pyramidal weakness. The impression was that the disease took a relapsing–remitting course, with sensory changes, pain and bladder symptoms being the most persistent symptoms. The patient had steroid therapy several times and she always reported improvement of symptoms after taking steroids. The patient's main complaints were pain affecting the arms and legs, frequency of micturation, pain in the jaw with inability to masticate food properly and vague gastrointestinal symptoms. The patient retired six years ago after her son died violently. The patient admitted being chronically depressed and she was on regular antidepressants.

Comments

A patient with a well-identified neurological condition is not immune from suffering from psychosomatic symptoms. Chronic conditions, whether they are neurological or secondary to other medical conditions such as bronchial asthma or coronary heart disease, are strongly influenced by the patient's emotional response to them. A model has been suggested in which the symptoms shown by a patient with a chronic disorder could be analysed in terms of the usual symptoms secondary to the neurological disorder and somatisation symptoms. The two sets could overlap, with frequent and alternating periods when one set of symptoms dominates the clinical picture depending on the activity of the primary disease on the one hand and the patient's psychosocial situation and his/her emotional reaction to it on the other.

The importance of utilising this model should not be underestimated, as it can guide the review process of the patient with a chronic condition and the formulation of an appropriate management plan according to the origin of the disabling presentation.

Somatisation is a diverse spectrum of symptoms, that are medically unexplained (Table 9.2). Such symptoms are extremely common and 25% of patients attending primary care services present with somatisation. The pathogenesis of somatisation symptoms is poorly understood. The prevailing view is that some people fail to express their distress in psychological or emotional terms and subsequently express their inner distress as physical symptoms.

Table 9.2. Common somatisation symptoms

Type	Symptoms
Pain	Diffuse pain, pain in extremities, back pain, headaches
Gastrointestinal	Nausea and vomiting, abdominal pain, diarrhoea, bloating
Cardiopulmonary	Palpitations, chest pain, shortness of breath
Neurological	Difficulty swallowing, loss of voice, deafness, double or blurred vision, fainting, dizziness, gait disturbance, seizures (pseudo-seizures), muscle weakness
Other	Fatigue, temporomandibular arthritis, burning sensations in the genitalia, dysparunia, dysmenorrhoea, irregular menstrual cycles, excessive menstrual bleeding

Differentiation between lower limb pain or pins and needles caused by somatisation or as a manifestation of the primary neurological condition can be difficult in a busy clinic. Knowledge of the social and vocational background can help in drawing the clinician's attention to the patients most likely to present with somatisation symptoms. A cluster of classic somatisation symptoms such as irritable bowel syndrome or temporomandibular joint arthritis can also raise the level of suspicion. Failure to respond to the standard treatment of a particular symptom is another red flag.

Failure to diagnose the somatisation syndrome as a co morbidity can lead to several problems, with unnecessary investigations, referrals and medications commonly arranged. The patient might not be in danger of increasing activity or severity of the primary disease but both disability and handicap are invariably compounded by the added anxiety and suffering.

Recognition of the role of somatisation in the way the patient presents should not be allowed to compromise the doctor–patient relationship, as the patient may start to have concerns about whether the doctor appreciates the seriousness of the symptoms. Therefore, strong reassurance about the nature of the symptoms should not be tainted by any change of the doctor's attitude towards the patient, stressing that the doctor still takes these problems very seriously.

Occasionally, some causes of the stress can be addressed. Organisation of voluntary work, respite care or marital counselling can address family tensions. Cognitive–behavioural therapy can often help people to deal with persistent unhelpful thoughts or behaviours. Symptomatic medical treatment is occasionally needed for symptoms such as nausea, diarrhoea or heartburn. Patients with associated mental health problems should be identified and managed appropriately.

Few patients will need formal psychological assessment and management. The standard approach to somatisation symptoms is the re-attribution model. The psychological input aims to help the patient to express distress and negative thoughts in psychological terms. Subsequently, this will lead to a reduction of the symptoms expressed physically. The re-attribution techniques should not necessarily be taught by a psychologist, as doctors or therapists could be trained in the basic principles of the therapy, enabling them to integrate the techniques into their routine work with the patients.

Further reading

Hilty, D. M., Bourgeois, J. A., Chang, C. H., Servis, M. E. (2001). Somatization disorder. *Curr Treat Opti Neurol* **3**, 305–320.

Pavlou, M., Stefoski, D. (1983). Development of somatizing responses in multiple sclerosis. *Psychother Psychosom* **39**, 236–243.

Complementary and alternative medicine

A 36-year-old woman with a five-year history of chronic fatigue syndrome and fibromyalgia asked if any method of complementary and alternative medicine (CAM) could help. She said that many of the people in the patients' support group had several therapies in the past, such as the Bowen technique, aromatherapy and crystal therapy. Most of the people were entirely satisfied with these therapies. She wants to know what is the best therapy for her condition

Comments

The triumph of modern scientific medicine is based on two pillars. Firstly, the anatomy and physiology of humans and the pathology of illness are extrapolated from scientifically sound investigations and this strong scientific foundation inspires different methods and interventions to manage illness. Secondly, the effect of any intervention is judged by stringent experiments that are designed to eliminate the effects of bias or placebo (double-blind, randomised controlled trials).

One would expect the other ways to promote healing that were popular in different areas around the world or originated from Europe centuries ago to completely vanish facing this overwhelming dominance of scientific medicine. Amazingly, the reverse has happened, with CAM gaining enormous popularity despite its failure to demonstrate its benefit unequivocally by the same strict analysis methodologies used to evaluate novel scientific medical interventions.

The reason for such success for CAM is simple: it works. Despite the continuous assault on CAM by the medical establishment, its popularity and utilisation is spreading mainly by word of mouth from satisfied patients.

It is impossible to evaluate CAM methods as one entity as the ideas and philosophies behind them vary greatly. Some authors define CAM as any medical practice that is outside the standard practice in a particular society. Consequently, acupuncture could hardly be considered as a CAM in China but biofeedback use in rehabilitation could be considered as a CAM in a country where it is rarely used. A more satisfactory definition includes all therapies where the basic ideas behind the therapy are not consistent with the current understanding of the way humans function as proposed by scientific medicine.

Many CAM therapies are based on the concept of energy. This theory considers well-being to be a state where the human's energy is balanced and illness is a state where such energy is unbalanced. It also proposes that such energy is channelled via Meridians and interventions targeting such meridians can restore the original balance. This concept is central to several CAMs such as acupuncture, reflexology, crystals and colour therapy and Reiki.

Other therapies such as aromatherapy and Ayveudic medicine use several herbs and essential oils to induce a therapeutic effect. Many of the substances used are proven to have pharmacological properties and it is not surprising to know that many patients find this approach useful, particularly for symptoms such as diffuse pain or stress.

Clinicians involved in rehabilitation research will probably be the most sympathetic to CAM practitioners, emphasising the difficulties of organising a methodologically robust experiment to evaluate a particular intervention. It is extremely difficult to blind a subject to an intervention such as a massage or physiotherapy technique. A reflexology session will not be very different from a sham reflexology session delivered to a control group. Most importantly, the attitude of a therapist carrying out a sham intervention is very difficult to control and to ensure it is as effective as the attitude of the other therapist delivering the genuine intervention.

Considering these difficulties, the lack of conclusive evidence of benefit of CAM could be explained by methodological difficulties or lack of funding to enable CAM research groups to design a trial with a sufficient number of subjects. Another explanation for the failure of CAM to demonstrate their effectiveness in randomised controlled trials is that they exert their effect mainly via a placebo effect. Placebo is known to be most effective when the intervention is delivered within a healing setting, with both therapist and patient believing in a solid rational behind the intervention. Frank and Frank (1991) proposed this concept when they tried to identify the main factors necessary for a successful psychotherapy intervention, stating: 'ritual or procedure that requires the active participation of both patient and therapist and that is believed by both to be the means of restoring the patient's health'.

Evaluation of meta-analyses of several CAM interventions seem to support such an idea, as these analyses suggest that the most important factor in the success or failure of a particular intervention is the therapist himself/herself, with the nature of the intervention having secondary importance. A good therapist is a charismatic person that is able through the healing setting to provide the patient with a psychic force that enables the patient to enhance his/her ability to promote healing.

Most patients seen in a rehabilitation setting, whether they have a neurological or a musculoskeletal condition or are suffering from a medically unexplained condition such as chronic fatigue syndrome or somatisation, will be invariably disappointed by the failure of the traditional medical methods to alter their illness. Many of them will have already tried or considered CAM as a way to improve their quality of life. It is important for rehabilitation clinicians to have a good idea about the types of CAM available so they can offer their

Table 9.3. Classification of complementary and alternative medicine

Proposed mode of action	Example
Biologically based therapies	Aromatherapy, dietary supplements
Manipulative and body based systems	Massage, osteopathy, Bowen technique
Alternative medical system	Homeopathy
Energy therapies	Acupuncture, reflexology, Reiki

patients an informed opinion and not just a point blank rejection of CAM as an option (Table 9.3). Ideally a rehabilitation service should have links to reputable local CAM practitioners so that recommendations could be made according to the patient's needs.

Reference

Frank, J. D., Frank, J. B. (1991). *Persuasion and Healing: A Comparative Study of Psychotherapy*, 3rd edn. Baltimore: Johns Hopkins University Press.

Further reading

Ernst, E. (2001). *The Desktop Guide to Complementary and Alternative Medicine: An Evidence-based Approach.* Edinburgh: Mosby.
Hyland, M. E. (2005). A tale of two therapies: psychotherapy and complementary and alternative medicine (CAM) and the human effect. *Clin Med* **5**, 361–367.

10

Spasticity management

Muscle spasticity is one of the few features of pyramidal paralysis that is relatively easy to manage pharmacologically and with different therapeutic modalities. Mild muscle spasticity can occasionally be beneficial to patients, for example to help with weight bearing. However, moderate and severe muscle spasticity usually necessitates prompt management as it is often associated with a combination of problems, such as painful spasms, general pain, postural instability, risk of joint contractures or problems with care provision to the patient.

Physiotherapy is the cornerstone of spasticity management in most instances. The medical assessment should include a general evaluation of potential factors that may contribute to the severity of the spasticity, such as urinary tract infections or pressure sores. The decision to initiate pharmacological therapy should always be discussed with the patient's physiotherapist, as reduction of muscle tone may impact on the physiotherapy programme. I usually encourage my physiotherapy colleagues to monitor the antispasticity drug dose titration as they are usually in the best position to monitor the medication's effects.

Management of spastic equinovarus deformity

A 62-year-old man with right hemiplegia presented with impaired mobility. He walked with a spastic circumducted gait and had difficulty clearing his right foot from the floor during the swing phase. Clinically, he had a right foot dynamic equinovarus deformity. Several options of management were discussed.

Comments

Spastic foot drop is a common cause of impaired mobility after upper motor neurone lesions. The pyramidally affected foot tends to drop rather than to go into dorsiflexion because the muscle spasticity secondary to such lesions predominantly affects the foot plantar flexors. The calf muscles are also anatomically bulkier and stronger than the foot dorsiflexors as they are responsible for stabilising the foot during standing and propelling the whole limb during the 'toe-off' movement at the end of the stance phase just prior to the leg swing. Spasticity of the gastrocnemius and soleus muscles leads to a continuous pull on the Achilles tendon, with subsequent loss of 'heel strike' in the start of the stance phase.

Spastic foot drop is often associated with a tendency of the foot to invert, leading to an equinovarus deformity. Increased muscle tone in the tibialis posterior muscle is the usual cause of equinovarus. Table 10.1 shows the main muscles implicated in the development of equinovarus. Both the tibialis anterior and the tibialis posterior are powerful foot invertors. However, the main action of the former is foot dorsiflexion while the latter is a plantar flexor. These actions can be seen during the normal gait cycle; tibialis anterior is normally active at heel strike and throughout the swing phase whereas tibialis posterior normally activates just after heel strike and stays active throughout the stance phase.

It is very important to assess the patient's gait carefully to determine the exact cause of the problem. Not all patients failing to clear their foot fully and scraping the floor during the swing phase of their gait have spastic plantar

Table 10.1. Muscles involved in equinovarus

	Gastrocnemius	Soleus	Tibialis anterior	Tibialis posterior
Origin	Back of femoral condyles	Posterior aspect of fibula and medial border of tibia	Interosseos membrane and upper half of lateral surface of the tibia	Interosseos membrane and posterior aspect of tibia and fibula
Insertion	Calcaneum (via Achilles tendon)	Calcaneum (via Achilles tendon)	Medial cuneiform bone	Navicular bone and medial cuneiform bone
Action	Plantar flexion	Plantar flexion and ankle stabilisation on standing	Dorsiflexion and inversion	Plantar flexion and inversion

flexors or weak dorsiflexors. Many of these patients will have profound muscle weakness in either hip or knee flexors, leading to failure to shorten the leg adequately during the swing phase. If gait assessment and clinical examination of the foot revealed either an equinus or an equinovarus deformity, the second step is to determine if the deformity is dynamic or fixed. A dynamic deformity can be passively corrected at rest. In most cases, the affected joint is dynamic to a certain degree but the examiner is unable to achieve the full range of movement of the ankle. It is important to try to determine when the spasticity stops and the soft tissue changes begin, as that degree of movement is often the one that could be achieved with appropriate management using methods such as stretching exercises, botulinum toxin injections or foot splints.

Dynamic equinus deformities can be managed by botulinum toxin injections into the gastrocnemius and soleus muscles. In equinovarus, the tibialis posterior should be injected as well. This is the deepest muscle on the back of the leg and is sandwiched between the flexor digitorum longus and the flexor hallucis longus. It is extremely difficult to inject the tibialis posterior accurately using surface anatomical markers and EMG or high-resolution ultrasound should be used to ensure exact placement of the injection. Tibialis posterior can be approached either anteriorly or posteriorly. Anterior approach is probably easier and more popular among those giving botulinum toxin injections.

Some patients present with ankle inversion as the main deformity, leading to an isolated varus deformity. The varus deformity causes the lateral aspect of the foot to strike the ground forcefully during the early part of the stance phase, leading to pain and occasional development of callosities at the outer aspect of the foot. Big toe extension during the early stance phase is a common association. This problem is usually caused by muscle spasticity in tibialis anterior with or without overactivity of the extensor hallucis longus. Botulinum toxin injection of tibialis anterior is relatively easy as it is a bulky muscle that can be palpated just lateral to the tibial chin.

In many cases, physiotherapy and pharmacological reduction of muscle tone are unable to maintain the range of movement in the affected joint and/ or improve the gait pattern and orthotic management is often needed. The AFO is the standard splint used in such patients. The prescription and type of AFO will depend on various factors. A fixed 'off the shelf' AFO could be used for an immobile patient needing simply to maintain the ankle's range of movement or to facilitate movement from sitting to standing. More rigid AFOs will be needed for patients who need to weight bear on the affected foot. Orthotic prescribers appreciate the fact that adjustments may be needed to shift the centre of gravity forwards and backwards according to the state of the proximal joints and the strength of the rest of the lower limbs in order to avoid creating significant moments working against a weak group of muscles.

Neuroprosthesis can also be used to manage patients with either equinus or equinovarus deformities. The most popular approach is to use functional electrical stimulation of the peroneal nerve. In a standard single-channel stimulation, a sensor in the patient's shoe detects 'heel rise' and sends an electrical impulse to a small device that can be attached to the patient's belt. This device triggers stimulation of the peroneal nerve, thus correcting foot drop in the swing phase. Patients can also be supplied with a multichannel functional electrical stimulator that stimulates different muscle groups such as foot dorsiflexors and knee flexors to try to achieve a better gait pattern. Functional electrical stimulation can be used for equinovarus deformities.

In most adults, surgical management is not needed. Children with spastic foot drop secondary to cerebral palsy might need surgical intervention, with procedures such as Achilles tendon lengthening to maintain mobility as the child grows up. In adults with varus deformities, transfer of an entire muscle (tibialis posterior or anterior) is occasionally indicated. Split muscle transfers can be performed, especially when the affected muscle is spastic in both stance and swing phases of gait. Fixed deformities can be managed surgically by procedures such as *osteotomy* or *arthrodesis.*

Further reading

Cioni, M., Esquenazi, A., Hirai, B. (2006). Effects of botulinum toxin-A on gait velocity, step length, and base of support of patients with dynamic equinovarus foot. *Am J Phys Med Rehabil* **85**, 600–606.

Kralj, A., Acimovic, R., Stanic, U. (1993). Enhancement of hemiplegic patient rehabilitation by means of functional electrical stimulation. *Prosthet Orthot Int* **17**, 107–114.

Management of generalised severe spasticity

A 34-year-old woman with a 12-year history of multiple sclerosis presented with severe spastic paraplegia. The patient was taking the full dosage of baclofen and dantrolene with very limited benefit. The patient could not tolerate tizanidine, diazepam or high doses of gabapentin. The patient complained bitterly that baclofen induced sedation, which was a particular problem as she was working part time. The patient's main complaint was of severe painful flexor and extensor lower limb spasms, which occasionally almost threw her out of her wheelchair.

Comments

Parapyramidal tracts refer to all the upper motor neurones that are not a part of the pyramidal tract. The term parapyramidal should not be confused with extrapyramidal, which is associated with the basal ganglia. Most of the parapyramidal tracts arise from the brainstem and are involved with the control of the spinal stretch, flexor and extensor reflexes. The dorsal reticulospinal tract (DRT), medial reticulospinal tracts (MRT) and the vestibulospinal tract (VST) have different roles. The DRT has a mainly inhibitory effect on the spinal reflexes while the MRT and VST stimulate the spinal reflexes.

Despite the fact that the three tracts originate from the brainstem, the DRT is the only one under cortical control. Therefore, a cortical lesion secondary to brain injury or stroke will affect mainly the DRT, with subsequent tipping of balance in favour of a more stimulatory drive. This phenomenon explains the tendency of cortical lesions to produce exaggerated spinal reflexes and muscle spasticity. The close proximity of the DRT to the pyramidal tract in the spinal cord make it more susceptible to injury in patients with spinal lesions leading to pyramidal weakness. The MRT and VST are located relatively distant to the pyramidal tract and are more likely to be spared, with the two tracts acting to stimulate the spinal stretch and extensor reflexes in such patients.

This strong association between upper motor neurone lesions, whether central or spinal, and muscle spasticity can be harmless or even occasionally useful, with some patients using the high muscle tone in their lower limbs to assist weight bearing on a weak leg. However, spasticity can result in significant clinical challenges in a large number of patients (Table 10.2). Clinicians use different methods to try to reduce the severity of muscle spasticity in order to achieve a particular goal, such as controlling painful spasms, or to try to prevent long-term damage to the joints.

Table 10.2. Some clinical problems associated with severe generalised spasticity

Painful muscle spasms
Non-specific pain
Joint contractures
Difficulty with maintaining hygiene
Difficulty with activities such as self-catheterisation
Problems with posture/seating
Pressure ulcers

Table 10.3. Commonly used antispasticity medications

Drug	Mode of action	Common side effects
Baclofen	GABA agonist	Sedation, dizziness, muscle weakness
Tizanidine	Agonist at α_2-adrenoceptors	Sedation, dizziness
Dantrolene	Inhibits release of intramuscular calcium stores	Impaired liver function
Diazepam	GABA agonist	Somnolence, dizziness, muscle weakness, addiction
Gabapentin	GABA agonist	Sedation, dizziness

GABA, γ-aminobutyric acid.

A multidisciplinary team of clinicians should ideally formulate a generalised spasticity management plan. The initial assessment should exclude any comorbidity that might worsen spasticity, such as pressure ulcers, chronic pain or infection. Identification of the spasticity-related problems and explicit goal setting should follow and a realistic management plan created. Patients may need pharmacological intervention, physical therapy, orthoses and/or equipment and aids. Good communication and timely interventions by the relevant members of the team are essential to facilitate the implementation of the management plan.

Most patients will respond to oral antispasticity medications (Table 10.3). Failure to tolerate higher doses of such drugs is not uncommon. Sedation is a particularly troublesome side effect, which in conjunction with the fatigue that patients with conditions such as multiple sclerosis may have can impact on the patient's functional abilities and quality of life.

Patients who fail to respond to or tolerate maximum doses of antispasticity medications present their treating clinicians with a difficult challenge. At this stage, re-evaluation of the clinical situation is essential to establish the main problems and to determine the need for further reduction of the muscle tone, as most of the options available at this stage are invasive and carry significant risk to the patient.

Traditionally, surgical rhizotomy and intrathecal phenol injections have proved to be very effective methods to treat generalised, severe lower limb spasticity. Anterior and posterior root rhizotomy aims to disrupt the spinal stretch reflexes and has been used for many years. The operation is irreversible and often affects urinary and faecal sphincteric control and sexual function. Several more-selective and less-destructive techniques to disrupt the reflex arch have been developed to try to avoid such serious complications. Intrathecal phenol injections might be a simpler procedure but it invariably leads to destruction of the autonomic control of the lower limbs, with a high risk of vasomotor disturbances and pressure ulcers. Sphincteric control is also lost. Phenol is now mainly used for peripheral nerve blocks.

Baclofen is probably the standard first-line oral medication used to reduce spasticity. Baclofen has poor penetration of the blood–brain barrier; consequently, a high oral dosage is required and side effects are common as most of the drug is metabolised peripherally without reaching its intended target. The intrathecal baclofen pump has been developed as a way to deliver the drug directly into the central nervous system, thus enabling a lower dosage and achieving a full pharmacological effect without the systematic side effects. The usual daily dose of intrathecal baclofen is approximately 200–400 µg, which is the equivalent of one 10 mg tablet a month.

The intrathecal pump is inserted surgically just beneath the anterior abdominal wall and its catheter is connected to the L3–L4 intrathecal space. The pump combines a reservoir and a delivery mechanism that is programmable to allow titration of the dose while the pump remains *in situ*.

The selection of the suitable patients for the pump is very important. Most patients using an intrathecal pump have severe, generalised lower limb spasticity that is not controlled with maximum doses of oral antispasticity medications. Patients with considerable contractures of the hips or knees are probably not suitable and patients with significant mental health or cognitive problems might find it difficult to cope with the whole procedure and with the refilling trips. Suitable candidates should be admitted to hospital for a trial in which a small dose of intrathecal baclofen is injected via a catheter and the response monitored. Patients responding well can proceed to the pump insertion.

Most patients need frequent reviews following pump insertion to adjust the baclofen dosage by reprogramming the pump. Once the optimum dose is determined, the patient need only be seen to refill the pump, which usually occurs every three to four months depending on the daily dose. These visits should be used to review the patient clinically as well as to ensure optimum control of spasticity with minimal side effects.

Problems with pump dysfunction, catheter kinking or disconnection are rarely seen now. However, problems with overdose or sudden withdrawal of baclofen are occasionally seen, most commonly because of human error in programming the pump or because of patients forgetting their refilling appointments.

Further reading

Sheean, G. (ed). (1998). *Spasticity Rehabilitation*. London: Churchill Communication, Europe.

Young, R. R. (1994). Spasticity: a review. *Neurology* **44** (Suppl. 9), S12–S20.

Penn, R. D., Savoy, S. M., Corcos, D., *et al.* (1989). Intrathecal baclofen for severe spinal spasticity. *N Eng J Med* **320**, 1517–1521.

11

Ventilatory support in rehabilitation

Injuries high in the cervical spine have traditionally been strongly associated with respiratory insufficiency and the occasional need for assisted ventilation. As the diaphragm is the prime respiratory muscle, disruption of its nerve supply through a spinal pathology or direct damage of the phrenic nerve, originating from C3–C5, can lead to serious respiratory failure. Cervical spine injuries sparing the phrenic nerve can still lead to significant respiratory insufficiency through interruption of the nerve supply to the different accessory respiratory muscles such as the abdominal and intercostal muscles.

A more common respiratory association with neurological disorders is sleep apnoea syndrome. Stroke can lead to the syndrome and conversely affected patients are more at risk of stroke. Despite the high prevalence of both conditions, this interesting relationship has not been adequately investigated and guidelines to screen stroke patients for sleep apnoea syndrome are lacking.

Artificial ventilation in Guillain–Barré syndrome

A 60-year-old man developed numbness in the feet following a diarrhoeal illness. He then developed weakness of his upper and lower limbs, which progressed slowly. Electrophysiology showed an axonal pattern of generalised neuropathy suggested by markedly reduced distal compound muscle action potentials and early denervation potentials in EMG. Examination of CSF confirmed the diagnosis of Guillain–Barré syndrome, and antibodies to *Campylobacter jejuni* were positive. The patient failed to respond to either immunoglobulin therapy or plasma exchange and within 10 days had paralysis of the respiratory muscles and cranial nerves and was admitted to intensive care, where he was intubated and ventilated.

Autonomic paralysis led to several problems, with labile blood pressure, arrhythmias and heart failure. He also had paralysis of the cranial nerves, leading to facial paralysis and ophthalmoplegia. The patient remained in intensive care for seven months. The patient's medical situation stabilised but his neurological condition showed no improvement. He remained dependent on ventilatory support. A meeting was called to discuss the prognosis and further management of the patient.

Comments

Respiratory failure is a well-recognized complication of Guillain–Barré syndrome and mechanical ventilation is required in 20–30% of patients. Hypoventilation is usually caused by respiratory muscle weakness, impaired bulbar function or both. The most important advance in the treatment of this disorder has been positive-pressure ventilation, which was developed during the European poliomyelitis epidemics of the 1950s. This has enabled patients with respiratory failure to survive until they recovered from paralysis.

The requirement for long-term respiratory support is unusual as most patients are weaned from assisted ventilation within three weeks of onset of Guillain–Barré syndrome. Nevertheless, a few patients require longer periods of assisted ventilation and their eventual recovery may be very slow. The management of this challenging group of patients is rarely reported and the final outcome could be underestimated as the follow-up in most of the studies has been limited to one year.

A few case reports describe the use of ventilation for up to one year. The longest period of assisted ventilation followed by successful weaning detailed in the literature is 22 months. Another patient needed nocturnal ventilation for five years before finally moving completely off assistance.

Where such patients should be managed is controversial. Most intensive care units are accustomed to patients with parynchymal pulmonary diseases or those who need surgical or postoperative respiratory care. It is unrealistic to expect these units to meet the needs of patients with respiratory muscle paralysis for long periods, especially to provide the rehabilitation and psychological aspects of management. Spinal injury units have the best facilities to address the complex issues such patients face. Where there will be a continuing need for ventilatory support in the community, spinal injury units will have the necessary experience to arrange smooth discharge plans as some of their patients have the same needs once in the community.

The same principles of rehabilitation used with patients with high cervical spine injuries requiring artificial ventilation could be implemented for patients with this syndrome. However, the patients' prolonged periods of artificial ventilation needed in Guillain–Barré syndrome can present unique rehabilitation challenges. Paralysis of the high cranial nerves is common, and this can make it very hard to establish reliable methods of communication. Eye blinking or movement is usually impaired, making it difficult for the patient to read or use communication aids. Special care should always be taken when caring for the eyes as exposure keratitis is not uncommon.

Persistent autonomic neuropathy can lead to ongoing problems with cardiac arrhythmias or labile blood pressure. The pattern of autonomic involvement in Guillain–Barré syndrome differs from that seen in spinal injuries, where the vagus nerve function is preserved (as it is a cranial nerve), thus leading to the parasympathetic drive taking the upper hand in the acute stage and the patient frequently needing regular anticholinergic blockade. In Guillain–Barré syndrome, the clinical impact of the persistent autonomic dysfunction is less predictable as both sympathetic and parasympathetic nerves are affected.

Maintaining range of movement in large joints can be more straightforward in patients with Guillain–Barré syndrome because there is no muscle spasticity. Special care should be given to prevent shortening of the Achilles tendon, which might complicate prolonged periods of foot drop while the patient is in bed. Physiotherapy and positioning are usually adequate to prevent this problem. Orthotic management might be needed in certain patients.

Bladder management is relatively easier in patients with Guillain–Barré syndrome than in patients with cervical spine injuries because flaccid paralysis of the bladder will facilitate catheterisation. The most serious bladder problems seen with spinal injuries, such as detruser/sphincter dyssynergia, do not occur in patients with Guillain–Barré syndrome.

Establishing the prognosis is extremely difficult in the acute stage. Nerve conduction studies indicate that a slower rate of recovery, usually 6 to 12 months, is associated with disease affecting axonal conduction. However, most clinicians dealing with patients requiring prolonged periods of ventilatory support will feel that the prognosis is generally poor and that the chances of recovery are extremely low. Nevertheless, it is important to emphasise to the patient the inadequacies in our knowledge and the variable long-term outcome.

Further reading

Chalmers, R. M., Howard, R. S., Wiles, C. M., et al. (1996). Respiratory insufficiency in neuronopathic and neuropathic disorders. Q J Med **89**, 469–476.

Fletcher, D. D., Lawn, N. D., Wolter, T. D., Wijdicks, E. F. M. (2000). Long-term outcome in patients with Guillain–Barré syndrome requiring mechanical ventilation. Neurology **54**, 2311–2315.

Diaphragmatic paralysis

A 44-year-old man presented with a five week history of shoulder and arm pain associated with upper limb weakness. The pain was very intense during the first two weeks but recently had become less intense. The patient had a severe viral illness two weeks before presentation. Clinical examination showed a patchy pattern of sensory loss and motor weakness and diagnosis of **neuralgic amyotrophy** was suggested. The patient was referred for rehabilitation.

On further assessment, the patient complained of shortness of breath when lying flat, which became more severe over two weeks. Clinically, he was noted to have a paradoxical chest and abdominal movement, with even greater respiratory distress when lying flat. There was a significant reduction in spirometry measures lying flat compared with standing, indicating a significant bilateral diaphragmatic weakness. Blood gases were consistent with type II respiratory failure with significant carbon dioxide retention and raised bicarbonate.

Comments

Neuralgic amyotrophy – also called amytrophic neuralgia, Parsonage–Turner syndrome or brachial neuritis – is a neurological condition that probably has an autoimmune pathology. The patient usually presents with severe pain affecting one or both shoulders and arms, which is followed by patchy sensory loss and motor weakness affecting the areas and muscles supplied by the brachial plexus but also sometimes affecting neighbouring nerves or nerve branches. A few weeks after presentation, the severity of pain starts to ease but several upper limb muscles show considerable atrophy. Nerve conduction studies often show loss of sensory and motor amplitudes with relatively normal conduction velocity and EMG shows denervation pattern in affected muscles.

Management of neuralgic amyotrophy is supportive with adequate analgesia and rehabilitation. Physical therapy should start as soon as the pain lessens in severity, with exercises aiming mainly at maintaining range of movements of the involved joints followed by strengthening exercises in the post-acute stage. Occupational therapy concentrates on hand function and equipment and aids to maximise independence. Most patients improve significantly within one to three years; however, a recent report has shown that almost two thirds of the patients continue to complain of either persistent pain or muscle weakness after three years.

Diaphragmatic paralysis is a recognised complication of neuralgic amyotrophy and can be unilateral or bilateral. Some authors suggested an incidence of diaphragmatic paralysis of up to 10–20% in such patients. Diaphragmatic paralysis can also follow other neurological conditions, such as multiple sclerosis, myopathies, muscle dystrophies and peripheral neuropathies.

The diaphragm is the most important respiratory muscle and is innervated by the cervical motor neurones C3–C5 via the phrenic nerves. During inspiration, diaphragm contraction creates more negative intrapleural pressure, with subsequent movement of air into the lungs.

In bilateral diaphragmatic weakness, the respiratory accessory muscles must do all the work of the breathing; however, when the patient is in a supine position, the paralysed diaphragm will allow the abdominal contents to be pushed into the chest, resulting in an increasing respiratory impairment. This will reduce vital capacity and total lung capacity, quite often by more than 50%, compared with a normal supine reduction of approximately 10%. Measurement of maximal inspirational pressure while supine can also show a significant reduction (up to $60\,cmH_2O$). Symptoms depend upon whether there is unilateral or bilateral paralysis and the presence or absence of any underlying pulmonary disease.

Typically, patients with bilateral diaphragmatic paralysis present with respiratory failure or dyspnoea and with worsening breathlessness on lying down. Occasionally this symptom is interpreted as orthopnoea and the patient is misdiagnosed as having a sign of heart failure. As a result of respiratory failure, a patient can present with insomnia, early morning headaches, excessive daytime somnolence and fatigue.

Clinical examination in bilateral diaphragmatic weakness reveals tachypnoea and excessive use of the accessory respiratory muscles. Chest examination reveals bilateral lower chest dullness with absent breath sounds but, most importantly, paradoxical inward movement of the abdomen with inspiration.

The prognosis of diaphragmatic paralysis depends upon the nature of the underlying disease. In neuralgic amyotrophy, recovery of diaphragmatic weakness usually lags behind upper limb recovery. However some patients show complete recovery of diaphragmatic function within two or three years.

The treatment of choice for symptomatic patients is non-invasive positive-pressure ventilation using a nasal or full-face mask, mainly at night for ambulatory patients. Positive-pressure ventilation via tracheostomy, either intermittent or permanent, may be required for patients with life-threatening diseases or a diagnosis of high tetraplegia.

Phrenic nerve pacing may be considered in patients who have intact phrenic nerve function and no evidence of myopathy. The ideal patient is one with high quadriplegia without intrinsic lung disease. A candidate for phrenic pacing will need comprehensive assessment including diaphragmatic EMG. The procedure is complex and patients with severe respiratory failure can use pacing in conjunction with other ventilatory methods mainly to facilitate community mobility without the need to carry bulky ventilatory equipments with them while outdoors.

Further reading

Hughes, P. D., Polkey, M. I., Moxham, J. (1999). Long term recovery of diaphragm strength in neuralgic amyotrophy. *Eur Respir J* **13**, 379–384.

van Alfen, N., van Engelen, B. G. M. (2006). The clinical spectrum of neuralgic amyotrophy in 246 cases. *Brain* **129**, 438–450.

12

Sphincteric dysfunction

Bladder, bowel and sexual impairments are strongly associated with neurological conditions. The impact of these impairments on the patient's quality of life cannot be underestimated. Bladder impairments are not only an inconvenient problem but can also lead to renal damage. Bowel impairment often inflicts more misery on patients but the problems are very rarely serious from a medical stand point.

Botulinum toxin for neuropathic bladder

A 36-year-old woman with a 12 year history of multiple sclerosis used tolterodine, intermittent catheterisation and intravesical oxybutinin to manage her neuropathic bladder but was still having several problems with urgency, frequency and occasional incontinence. The patient is not keen on either a urethral or a suprapubic catheter as she is sexually active.

Comments

A standard bladder management plan aims mainly to achieve two goals: maintaining a safe, low-pressure system and ensuring continence. It will not always be possible to achieve the two goals and a balance between them must be struck.

A simple way to understand the neuroanatomy of the urinary bladder is to consider its two main muscle types.

The **detrusor muscle** is a smooth muscle that lies in the wall of the bladder. It is mainly controlled by autonomic innervation through a cholinergic parasympathetic supply originating from S2–S4 roots. This stimulates muscarinic muscle receptors in the wall of the bladder to cause bladder contraction and urine voiding.

The **external urethral sphincter** comprises voluntary striated muscle innervated by the pudendal nerve, a somatic supply originating from the S2–S4 roots. Contraction of the sphincter closes the bladder outlet and maintains continence.

The **internal sphincter** and the **bladder neck** connect the detrusor muscle to the external sphincter and form an area rich in alpha-adrenoceptors. Sympathetic stimulation of these receptors originates mainly from T11–T12 roots and leads to internal sphincter contraction and further maintenance of continence.

In normal subjects, the whole system works in synergy. The default situation is of detrusor muscle relaxation, allowing the bladder reservoir to fill, and internal and external sphincter contraction to maintain continence. Parasympathetic stimulation will cause detrusor contraction and is accompanied by sympathetic inhibition to allow sphincteric relaxation and subsequent micturition.

Most patients with a neurological disorder will have neurogenic bladders caused by either upper or lower motor neurone lesions. Conditions affecting mainly the central nervous system such as stroke, brain injury, Parkinson's disease or multiple sclerosis usually lead to upper motor neurone lesions and a hyper-reflexic overactive bladder with a subsequent inability to store urine. As parasympathetic nerves provide the main stimulus leading to detrusor muscle contraction, selective anticholinergic drugs are the standard first-line management for such condition. It is unusual to try to stimulate the sympathetic alpha-adrenoceptors in the internal sphincter/bladder neck region with adrenergic agents as such drugs are usually poorly tolerated and their effectiveness is rather limited.

Botulinum toxin injection of the detrusor muscle has proved a valuable tool in refractory conditions with hyperactive bladders. The procedure is relatively simple and can be performed as a day case procedure. The botulinum toxin is diluted in normal saline and injected through a cystoscope. As in injections to skeletal muscles, it is very difficult to predict the outcome and patients vary greatly. Most patients will have a therapeutic benefit that lasts for more than six months. Repeat injections can then be arranged accordingly. Some patients with problems with pain from a catheter or by-passing owing to a hyper-reflexic bladder can benefit from intravesical botulinum toxin.

Conditions such as cauda equina or autonomic neuropathy usually lead to a flaccid hypotonic bladder with or without bladder outlet tightness. The patient usually has chronic retention with overflow. Alpha blockers can occasionally help to relax the internal sphincter and facilitate more efficient bladder emptying. Intermittent catheterisation is very valuable in most patients as it helps to achieve complete bladder emptying, thus preventing urine stagnation and increased risk of infections or stone formation.

Injecting botulinum toxin into the external urethral sphincter in patients with hypoactive bladder and sphincteric tightness has been shown to reduce the post-void urinary residual volume. A major advantage of this procedure is the very low incidence of sphincteric incompetence, which is a common complication following surgical resection of the urethral sphincter – once a popular approach to manage such a difficult problem.

Many conditions lead to detrusor–sphincter dyssynergia, when both detruser and sphincter contracting simultaneously, leading to a massive increase in the intravesical pressure and infected urine ascending to the kidneys. Up to 80% of patients with spinal cord injuries may have detrusor–sphincter dyssynergia. In the 1950s, chronic renal failure used to be the leading cause of death in patients surviving the acute stage of spinal cord injury. Renal failure usually followed sustained high intravesical pressures and large bladder residues, resulting in upper tract damage. Now, thanks to the increased understanding of the mechanism of the urological complications of spinal injuries, that risk is substantially reduced but all patients with a spinal cord injury should have an annual urological review and aggressive management of any abnormalities.

The appropriate investigation in an annual review for the asymptomatic patient depends on its sensitivity and specificity. The test does not have to be specific but it needs to be highly sensitive in order to detect the earliest signs of renal involvement. Renograms using radioactive isotopes are non-specific but they are highly sensitive; consequently, these are the standard screening test used. Patients with abnormal renograms and symptomatic patients usually have renal ultrasound and plain radiography, which are not only safe and non-invasive but are also excellent in picking up structural abnormalities in the renal system, including renal stones.

To diagnose detrusor–sphincter dyssynergia, urodynamic studies will be needed to give a detailed picture of the behaviour of the lower urinary tract and identify risk factors such as high-pressure storage. The results can then inform an appropriate management plan.

The role of botulinum toxin in the management of this problem is not certain. Several studies have shown the effectiveness of intraperineal urethral injection of botulinum toxin in patients with spinal cord injuries. A recent trial had to be stopped prematurely as patients with multiple sclerosis and detrusor–sphincter dyssynergia receiving intravesical botulinum toxin showed no improvement in relation to placebo-injected controls. However, as the use of botulinum toxin to manage neuro-urological impairments become more popular, the exact indications, technique and potential problems will become clearer.

Further reading

Smith, C.P., Somogyi, G.T., Boon, T.B., *et al.* (2004). Botulinum toxin in urology: evaluation using an evidence based medicine approach. *Nat Clin Pract Urol* **1**, 31–37.

De Seze, M., Petit, H., Gallien, P., *et al.* (2002). Botulinum toxin and detruser sphincter dysynergia: a double blind lidocaine controlled study in 13 patients with spinal cord injuries. *Eur Urol* **42**, 56–62.

Gallien, P., Reymann, J.M., Amareaco, G. (2005). Placebo controlled randomised double blind study of the effects of botulinum A toxin on detruser sphincter dysynergia in multiple sclerosis. *J Neurol Neurosurg Psychiatry* **76**, 1670–1676.

Schurch, B., Stohrer, M., Kramer, G., *et al.* (2000). Botulinum-A toxin for treating detrusor hyperreflexia in spinal cord injured patients: a new alternative to anticholinergic drugs? Preliminary results. *J Urol* **164**, 692–697.

Bowel dysfunction following spinal injury

A 34-year-old man with a T6 complete spinal injury has been having many problems managing his bowels. He is on a twice a week bowel management programme using glycerine suppositories before the programme and senna the night before. He has experimented with several laxatives but found that most of them led to frequent and unpredictable attacks of incontinence. His bowel programme has become difficult to perform because of his haemorrhoids and he is almost always in discomfort because of either constipation or incontinence.

Comments

A spinal injury specialist once said: 'If a spinal injury patient died a few weeks after injury, it is probably a pulmonary embolism. If he died years after the injury, it is probably renal failure. But if he committed suicide, it is probably bowel dysfunction.'

This statement reflects the misery that bowel dysfunction can create and applies to patients with neurological disorders affecting the innervation of the lower gut as well as to those with spinal injuries. Impaired mobility, swallowing difficulties and poly-pharmacy may also contribute to the difficulties patients have maintaining normal bowel function. In spinal injury, several gastrointestinal disorders such as gastro-oesophageal reflux, cholecystitis, pancreatitis and superior mesenteric artery syndrome are more common than in the normal population.

Most of the gastrointestinal tract is under involuntary control, with several central and local mechanisms controlling motility and function. Autonomic control is instrumental in maintaining normal bowel function, with the vagus nerve providing the main parasympathetic supply. The sympathetic supply originates from thoracic levels T4–T12 with the hypogastric nerve branching to form the superior mesentric and ciliac ganglia. The vagus and hypogastric nerves supply the gut down to the transverse colon. The rest of the colon, rectum and anus receive their parasympathetic supply from S2–S4 and their sympathetic supply from L1–L3, making this area very vulnerable to any spinal injury however low the level. The external sphincter is the only area of the lower gut under voluntary control. It is supplied by S2–S4 via the pudendal nerve. The external anal and pelvic muscles are in a state of continuous contraction even during sleep, thus maintaining faecal continence.

In normal subjects, reflex migratory contractions advance stool to the rectum. The internal sphincter then relaxes, allowing the stool to extend the rectum thus generating a conscious urge. The internal sphincter has a rich sensory nerve supply allowing accurate awareness of the nature of the rectal material, thus allowing gases to be passed when socially convenient and soft or hard stool to be voided when appropriate. Relaxation of the external anal sphincter and simultaneous contraction of the levator ani, abdominal muscles and diaphragm elevate intra-abdominal pressure and propel the stool out.

The complexity of this process makes it easy to appreciate the difficulty a neurologically impaired patient may face in controlling bowel function, with constipation, incontinence and poor coordination commonly seen. The pattern of bowel dysfunction in neurological disorders depends on the location of the lesion. Patients with upper motor neurone lesions will have a significantly different presentation from patients with lower motor neurone lesions (Table 12.1). Bowel dysfunction caused by upper motor neurone lesions is relatively easier to manage as normal bowel reflexes, such as the gastrocolic reflex and the anorectal reflex, are usually intact and can be used to establish a regular bowel management programme.

Constipation is an almost universal symptom in immobile patients with a neurological disorder. Its management is very difficult in patients who suffer from recurrent faecal incontinence, as most of the standard advice given to constipated patients can lead to incontinence, which most patients find more distressing than the constipation itself. Increasing fibre and fluid intake can help many patients but can also worsen the situation for others; therefore, a personalised management programme has to be designed for each patient. Assessment of the patient should start with documenting a food/fluid diary and a bowel habit diary and revision of the patient's medications, lifestyle and

Table 12.1. Bowel dysfunction with upper and lower motor neurone lesions

	Upper motor neurone	Lower motor neurone
Causes	Central: stroke Spinal injuries, multiple sclerosis	Cauda equina, e.g. disc prolapse Autonomic neuropathy, e.g. diabetes mellitus, Guillain–Barré syndrome
Pathology	Overactive segmental peristalsis, underactive propulsive peristalsis, hyperactive holding reflex with anal constriction	Reduced peristaltic movements, slow propulsion, low anal tone, absent gastrocolic and anorectal reflexes
Clinical picture	Chronic constipation	Severe constipation with overflow diarrhoea
Management	Standard bowel programme, sacral root stimulator	Stool softeners, frequent bowel evacuation to avoid overflow, manual evacuation

Table 12.2. General principles in management of constipation

Review medications, e.g. anticholinergic drugs, baclofen and
  tizanidine worsen constipation
Encourage fluid intake to at least 1.5–2 litres/day
Encourage fibre intake
Review defecation process
If stools are hard, consider stool softeners or osmotic preparations,
  e.g. lactulose
If stools are soft, consider stimulating medications, e.g. senna

toilet facilities, including the availability of carers and the patient's position while opening the bowels. Advice needs to combine general principles to manage constipation (Table 12.2) and specific advice based on information acquired during the assessment.

A standard bowel programme should aim at a daily bowel motion; however, most patients eventually establish a programme of two or three times a week. The bowel programme uses the gastrocolic reflex around an hour after breakfast or dinner with or without the use of glycerine suppositories or other laxatives. Particular attention should be paid to the patient's posture when trying to open the bowels. The anorectal reflex can be stimulated by digital stimulation of the rectum. Some patients will have refractory bowel dysfunction and manual evacuation or regular enemas will be needed.

Some patients with upper motor neurone lesions may be suitable for a sacral root stimulator device to control their bladder and bowel function.

The device uses electrical stimulation with different frequencies to stimulate either smooth muscles such as the detrusor muscle or striated muscles such as the external anal sphincter. The surgical procedure starts with a dorsal rhyzotomy for afferent roots S2–S4; this is followed by insertion of electrodes to stimulate the sacral anterior roots. Most patients report improvement in their bladder and bowel function and some are also able to produce penile erections using the device.

Comfort and continence are not always achieved using a standard bowel programme. The bowel programme could also be difficult to perform because of other factors such as the presence of haemorrhoids or the risk of autonomic dysreflexia. Clinicians should not shy away from discussing a *colostomy* with the patient once they have exhausted all non-surgical strategies to manage their patient's bowels effectively. Surprisingly, most patients report dramatic improvement of their quality of life following a colostomy. Suitable candidates should have preoperative transit time studies to determine the level of the procedure. If the studies show that stool accumulates in the rectosigmoid, a sigmoid colostomy should be performed. An ileostomy will be needed if transit studies indicate an atonic colon.

Further reading

Coggrave, M., Wiesel, P. H., Norton, C. (2006). Management of faecal incontinence and constipation in adults with central neurological diseases. *Cochrane Database Syst Rev* **3**, CDOO2115.

Weingarden, S. W. (1992). The gastrointestinal system and spinal cord injury. *Phys Med Rehabil Clin North Am* **3**, 765–779.

13

Communication disabilities

The statement that 'more than 80% of communication is non-verbal' is often made by clinicians when reassuring patients with communication problems owing to neurological disorders concerning the prognosis and prospects for social and vocational activities. The statement aims also at preparing the patient to accept the philosophy of their speech and language rehabilitation programme, which relies heavily on teaching the patient new strategies to cope with their disabilities. Many patients find it difficult to accept this rational and insist on therapy efforts directed mainly to restoring normal speech.

Unfortunately, there is no evidence that any therapy intervention can improve the quality of speech in dysphasic patients. However, implementing different compensatory strategies has been shown to reduce the patient's handicap and improve their quality of life.

Expressive aphasia

A 68-year-old man had a stroke leading to right hemiplegia. His speech was severely affected and became very laboured. He responded appropriately to commands but found it very difficult to speak in sentences and resorted to saying a few single words to try to express himself. The patient could also obey written commands but was unable to write even his name.

Comments

The main cognitive impairments resulting from dominant hemisphere damage are **aphasia** and **apraxia** (the terms dysphasia and dyspraxia are interchangeable with aphasia and apraxia). Aphasia is defined as impairment of language function caused by brain damage. **Mutism** is a complete failure of speech output, which can be congenital or acquired. Mutism can follow any severe language or articulation disorder. It can also be seen in patients with mental health conditions.

Two major centres in the dominant hemisphere control language function. Wernicke's area is located in the posterior superior part of the temporal lobe and is involved mainly with comprehension. Language output is primarily controlled by Broca's area in the inferior aspect of the fronatal lobe. These areas are connected by the arcuate fasciculus.

There are many classifications of aphasia syndromes. The most clinically useful one divides aphasia into two main categories: fluent and non-fluent (Fig. 13.1). As a rule of thumb, patients with fluent aphasia will have damage to Wernicke's or surrounding areas, while patients with non-fluent aphasia will have damage to Broca's or surrounding areas. Most patients will have a clinical picture that is mixed with elements of both syndromes. Clinicians should try to determine the dominant features of the communication disorder and then establish the diagnosis, prognosis and management plan accordingly. For example, almost all patients with aphasia will have *nominal* impairment 'inability to name objects'. But the term **nominal aphasia** should only be used when patients present with difficulties in naming objects as the

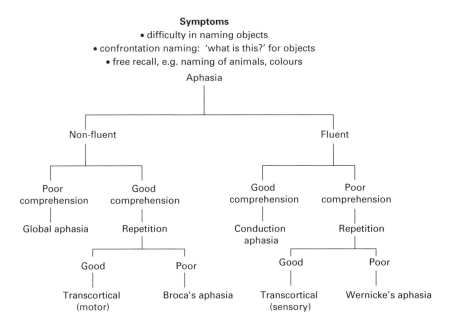

Figure 13.1 A flow chart for the diagnosis of aphasia. (Adapted from Goodglass *et al.*, 2001.)

most prominent feature of their communication impairment. The term **global aphasia** could be used to describe a patient with almost equal elements of aphasia.

Some patients retain an excellent ability to repeat spoken words or complex sentences despite having profound fluent or non-fluent aphasia. It was thought that a direct pathway exists between auditory centres and verbal motor centres, by-passing the damaged language centres and so the term **transcortical aphasia** was proposed. That theory was disproved but the term has remained. Transcortical aphasia can be either motor or sensory. In the motor form, the lesion is in the dominant lobe anterior and superior to Broca's area. Patients with this lesion present similarly to those with lesions of Broca's area but they retain an excellent ability to repeat even complex sentences. The lesion responsible for transcortical sensory aphasia is located on the border of the dominant parietal and temporal lobes. Patients with lesions here have good ability to repeat sentences without being able to understand their meaning.

The severity of non-fluent aphasia ranges between mutism to mild word-finding difficulties. In its milder form, non-fluent aphasia could sound fluent enough. The lack of grammar, paraphasias (mistaken words) and the intact comprehension abilities are indicative of non-fluent aphasia. Impairment of writing ability (agraphia) usually mirrors the spoken language in Broca's aphasia. Ability to read out loud is also impaired, with retained ability to understand written words.

Most patients with non-fluent aphasia will have good insight into their disability and are usually keen to participate in therapy. After assessment, realistic goals should be set. Many patients will have achieving normal speech as their main goal. That might not be a realistic goal and further negotiations should take place to try to formulate goals that are potentially achievable. It should be made clear to the patient and the family that improving *communication* should be the ultimate goal rather than just speech. Therefore, a rehabilitation programme can concentrate on either improving speech using methods such as repetitions, reading, melodic intonation therapy, syntax stimulation programmes or on using compensatory methods for communication such as visual charts, drawing boards or communication aids.

Communication aids can be initially difficult for patients to accept and some of them consider their use to be a form of *giving up* on their speech, while others will have concerns that continuing use of communication aids might impede their speech recovery process. Communication aids will be most useful for patients with severe expressive aphasia with almost intact comprehension and cognitive functions. Nowadays, it is not necessary to provide patients with bulky aids and there are simple software programmes that could be installed in mobile phones, thus enabling patients to communicate easily. Such an approach might be very useful with young patients,

Table 13.1. Apraxia

Type of apraxia	Assessment/command	Localisation
Orobuccal	Lick you lips Pretend to blow a match	Left inferior frontal lobe
Ideomotor	Pretend that you are hammering a nail to the wall Pretend that you are combing your hair	Parietal or frontal lobes
Ideational	Pretend that you are making a cup of tea Pretend that you are opening a letter	Corpus callosum

who will already have adequate knowledge of contemporary electronic devices and gadgetry.

Because apraxia is caused by lesions anatomically close to Broca's area, it is a common clinical association with aphasia. Rarely, apraxia can be the main cause of aphasia. In general, the presence of apraxia as a copathology in aphasic patients is a very poor prognostic factor and it is, therefore, important to identify patients with apraxia. In patients with intact comprehension, the diagnosis is relatively straightforward. Apraxic patients will have difficulty performing simple tasks involving moving the lips or tongue or involving the use of oral muscles, such as licking the lips or whistling to command. Clinicians should note that the three main types of apraxia rarely coexist (Table 13.1) as the affected brain centres responsible for each type are distinct. It is also interesting that many descriptions such as dressing apraxia or construction apraxia are not related to the genuine apraxic syndromes and they are mainly caused by separate pathologies such as unilateral neglect.

Reference

Goodglass, H., Kaplan, E., Barresi, B. (2001). *Boston Diagnostic Aphasia Examination*, 3rd edn. New York: Lippincott, Williams & Wilkins.

Further reading

Caplan, D. (1987). *Neurolinguistics and Linguistic Aphasiology: An Introduction.* New York: Cambridge University Press.
Hodges, J. R. (1994). *Cognitive Assessment for Clinicians.* Oxford: Oxford University Press.

Jargon aphasia

A 42-year-old woman made an excellent physical recovery from an attack of herpes simplex encephalitis. Three months later, she continued to have considerable problems with her speech, which was fluent but confused plus what appeared to be poor comprehension and inappropriate words and responses.

Comments

In aphasia, there is a breakdown of the three main components of language: phonology, semantics and syntax (Table 13.2). In pure Wernicke's aphasia, pathology is located in the superior temporal lobe in the dominant hemisphere. The clinical picture is usually consistent with the anatomical localisation of these three main components of language, with phonology and semantics significantly impaired and the syntax relatively preserved. Patients with Wernicke's aphasia will have fluent speech with relatively preserved grammar (syntax) but substantially impaired substance and content. There are very few information conveying words or nouns (semantics) and several paraphasias. Speech is effortless and the patient usually has poor insight into any difficulty. Comprehension and naming are always impaired.

Patients with isolated damage to the arcuate fasciculus, which anatomically joins Broca's and Wernicke's areas, will suffer from **conduction aphasia**.

Table 13.2. Basic language functions

Language function	Character	Impairment	Location
Phonology	Production and comprehension of appropriately sequenced speech sounds (phonemes)	Phonemic paraphasia, e.g. *cane* instead of *crane*	Left superior temporal lobe
Semantic	Production and comprehension of linguistically appropriate individual words	Semantic paraphasia, e.g. *table* instead of *desk*	Left temporal lobe
Syntax	Assembly of words into proper sentences	Agrammatism, e.g. *I stroke year* instead of *I had a stroke last year*	Left anterior hemisphere

This rare type of fluent aphasia is similar to Wernicke's aphasia but with two significant differences. In conduction aphasia, comprehension is relatively preserved but phonemic abilities are very limited, leading to frequent paraphasias, for example clean instead of clear. Repetition is usually severely affected in conduction aphasia.

The main challenge that clinicians face when dealing with a patient with fluent but incoherent and confused speech is to determine if the primary problem is mainly linguistic or if it is a result of other forms of cognitive impairment. All aphasic patients have naming problems. Therefore, a first step in the diagnosis of aphasia is to establish the presence of a naming disorder (anomia). Patients will have different degrees of difficulty and many will have anomia relevant to a specific semantic category such as colours. Confrontation naming (i.e. 'What is this?') may be easier than free recall (e.g. name as many body parts as possible). Considering the importance of naming in establishing the diagnosis of aphasia, clinicians should test it in the most comprehensive way using several objects for both confrontation naming and free recall.

Patients with primary diffuse cognitive impairment will have relatively intact language components, with infrequent paraphasias. The speech in general will have more substance and content. However, this content might be inappropriate, with disorientation and occasional confabulations rather than paraphasias. Comprehension is usually impaired in fluent dysphasics, whose answers will indicate almost complete misunderstanding of the questions asked. Confused or disorientated patients will show better understanding of questions or demands. Patients with pure communication disorders will often exhibit normal body language and eye contact, while patients with more generalised cognitive impairment will be more easily distracted and may demonstrate inappropriate responses.

In conditions causing diffuse brain damage such as traumatic brain injury, subarachnoid haemorrhage or encephalitis, patients present with mixed features of cognitive and linguistic disorders, especially in the early stages. Patients might be mute for weeks or months; this is caused not just by cognitive and language impairments but also by complex problems with articulation and phonation. The combination of these disturbances has become known as 'generalised deficits of cognition' and the treatment offered is, therefore, 'cognitive rehabilitation'. As recovery continues, distinct cognitive impairments will become more evident. It is then important to try to establish the main components of the cognitive impairment in order to formulate a beneficial rehabilitation programme.

Patients with more localised brain damage (e.g. stroke) usually have more clear-cut cognitive impairments, and attempts to identify the main components of the cognitive function could reveal distinct cognitive or linguistic syndromes. Some patients suffering a stroke will already have a background of cognitive impairment, for example dementia. Premorbid history may help to establish the extent of the cognitive impairment prior to the current illness.

Two factors make rehabilitation of fluent aphasics more challenging than non-fluent aphasics: lack of insight and poor comprehension. These substantially impede the patient's participation. A detailed assessment should identify the severity of the impairment and how it contributes to the patient's activities and participation. Patients with moderately severe fluent aphasia could find it difficult to participate because of lack of insight. Rehabilitation should concentrate on the patient's family and carers. When communicating with the patient, carers should talk slowly, use short and simple sentences and use gestures and body language to enhance and clarify the message. A picture book can also be used to indicate the basic needs for the patient such as meals or using the toilet.

Milder forms of aphasia can leave reading ability relatively intact and/or retain modest auditory comprehension skills. A corpus of words with their pictorial presentations should be presented to patients to read loudly and the exercise repeated. The aim is to concentrate on a relatively few important words that the patient can use accurately either when talking or when listening. This approach should ultimately make patients aware of their errors, especially with paraphasias. Some patients find this approach very demanding and exhausting. Ironically, a successful conclusion of this stage of rehabilitation may turn an incoherent but fluent speech to a more coherent but less-fluent speech and generate a more frustrated patient.

Eventually, many patients will end up with better speech quality that is less fluent. Some patients will find the whole process stressful, especially patients with moderate impairment as their lack of insight makes it difficult to motivate themselves. Family and carers are occasionally very keen on achieving some improvement regardless of how distressing the process can become.

Further reading

Helm-Eastabrooks, N., Albert, M. L. (1991). *Manual of Aphasia Therapy*. Austin, TX: Pro-Ed.

Hypokinetic dysarthria

A 69-year-old man was referred for speech and language therapy for problems with his speech. The patient was in the early stages of Parkinson's disease.

His speech difficulties were mildly disabling. There was some reduction in his speech intelligibility. He reported that requests for repetitions when he was speaking were more frequent and that communication was more difficult in noisy situations.

Comments

Speech is a complex behaviour that requires the coordinated contraction of a large number of muscles for its production. Control of the function of these muscles occurs via complex upper and lower motor pathways with considerable input from other neurological areas such as the cerebellum and basal ganglia. Impairment of the function of any of these neurological areas can lead to a specific problem affecting the speech articulation (Table 13.3)

Dysarthria is a specific speech disorder in which the muscles controlling articulation, respiration, phonation, prosody and resonation are affected (Table 13.4). Hypokinetic dysarthria is caused by problems with the extrapyramidal system. Almost 70% of patients with Parkinson's disease report that speech and voice are affected after their disease onset. Most of these speech difficulties are caused by hypokinetic dysarthria.

The clinical presentation of hypokinetic dysarthria in Parkinson's disease is consistent with the underlying pathology. Phonation changes may result from rigidity of the laryngeal musculature, and imprecise articulation and fast rate of speech usually reflect rigidity of the speech muscles. Bradykinesia can cause inappropriate silences and difficulty initiating speech movements. Lack of facial expression is also likely to be caused by bradykinesia.

Speech therapy aims at teaching new skills to these patients to improve their speech. Changing speech habits and bringing speech under voluntary control requires time and effort and a commitment to a practice routine. The most successful candidates for therapy with mild dysarthria are those who are highly motivated and for whom speech is an important aspect for daily living.

Table 13.3. Common types of dysarthria

Type	Localisation	Common causes
Hypokinetic	Basal ganglia	Parkinson's disease
Hyperkinetic	Basal ganglia	Dystonia, tremors, athetosis
Flaccid	Lower motor neurone	Bulbar palsy
Spastic	Upper motor neurone	Pseudobulbar palsy (motor neurone disease)
Ataxic	Cerebellum and its connections	Multiple sclerosis

Table 13.4. Process of human speech

Process	Comments
Respiration	Expiration of the air through the vocal mechanism is the energy source of audible speech
Phonation	Voice produced by modification of the air stream as it passes through the subglottic region; contraction of the subglottic muscles raises pressure and increases voice intensity
Resonation	Resonance within the pharyngeal, oral and nasal cavities modifies and amplifies the raw vocal tone
Articulation	Coordinated action of the tongue, lips, jaw and soft palate regulates the air stream and produces meaningful sounds (phonems)
Prosody	Melody, pauses, intonation and accents that enhance and enliven speech are mainly controlled by centres in the non-dominant hemisphere

A standard therapy programme focuses on increasing respiratory support, increasing phonatory effort to improve voice volume, increasing pitch variability and reducing the rate of speech. Most patients need 6–12 therapy sessions with commitment to practise the new learned skills at home and in everyday activities. Most patients achieve significant improvement by the end of the programme, being able to speak louder with reduction of speech rate and improved ability to articulate. This generates improvement of the overall intelligibility of speech.

Patients with mild dysarthria caused by Parkinson's disease are not consistently referred for speech intervention. Speech and language therapy referrals typically come late in the progression of the disease after dysarthria has become severe. Early referrals and prompt intervention are beneficial as even mild dysarthria can have functional limitations. Quality of speech is especially critical for those with heavy communication demands in their work.

Learning good speaking habits is easier in the early stages of the condition than waiting until symptoms are so severe that learning new skills is difficult. Learning to adjust and speak more clearly early will also help to maintain skills as the disease progresses and might also prevent depression and social isolation.

Further reading

Hartelius, L., Svensson, P. (1994). Speech and swallowing symptoms associated with Parkinson's disease and multiple sclerosis: a survey. *Fol Phoniatr Logopaed* **46**, 9–17.

Mutch, W. J., Strudwick, A., Roy, S. K., Downie, A. W. (1986). Parkinson's disease: disability, review, and management. *Br Med J* **293**, 675–677.

14

Sensory disability

Visually impaired patients are usually supported by specialised rehabilitation teams (e.g. sensory disability teams in the UK) and new technology has enabled patients to have a better quality of life. Equipment such as hand-held satellite navigation devices can allow patients to mobilise with much more ease in the community. Special software can convert written Internet pages to spoken words. Even the colour of shirts and ties can be detected using another useful device.

Visual impairment in neurologically impaired patients has a much more devastating effect. The visual impairment can be mild but in conjunction with the other physical, cognitive or behavioural disabilities, it can lead to a more challenging handicap. The visual impairment often has an unusual cause and this leads to a unique sensory problem. A severely ataxic patient can suffer from oscillopsia, which not only affects vision but also affects balance. Another patient with cortical blindness may be able to read small print but is unable to recognise his wife's face. These unusual problems are extremely difficult to address and a standard sensory disability team will often lack experience with such rare presentations.

Rehabilitation of such patients is best implemented jointly, with the patient's neurological rehabilitation team working with the sensory disability team. The neurological rehabilitation team will possess the necessary skills in assessment and management of the cognitive and physical problems while the sensory team can advise about issues such as home adaptations, access to services and special equipment.

Cortical blindness

A 72-year-old man was admitted to hospital with sudden collapse. A CT scan showed a massive haemorrhagic stroke affecting mainly the occipital lobes. The patient had a history of hypertension. He slowly regained consciousness but was very confused and aggressive. Four days later, and by the time the patient regained his mobility, it was clear to the staff that the patient was unable to see. Visual examination was difficult but the anterior chambers of both eyes and retinas looked normal and the pupillary reflexes were intact.

The patient had bizarre behaviour and he clearly had visual hallucinations reflecting incidents from his time in the army. The episodes of confusion and visual hallucinations were separated by periods when the patient appeared more lucid and rational. However, he remained disorientated and a formal psychological assessment was deemed too demanding for the patient as it might precipitate further confusion.

Three weeks after the stroke, the patient remained confused and the visual hallucinations persisted. He could not differentiate between light and dark and he had an inverted sleep rhythm with wandering and aggression at night.

The patient's family were very distressed and they wanted to discuss the plan of management and prognosis.

Comments

The visual cortex lies in the occipital part of the brain and constitutes about 20% of the cerebral cortex in humans. Structurally, it can be subdivided into six layers. The primary visual cortex, or area V1 (also known as striate cortex), is the primary target of fibres (axons) originating from the retina. Area V1 contains a topographic map of visual space. The extrastriate cortex comprises areas V2–V6. The striatal and extrastriatal areas interact in a very complex way to interpret the colour, shape and movement of visual images.

Cortical blindness refers to loss of vision following bilateral occipital cortex lesions. Hemispheric lesions do not reduce visual acuity but instead lead to peripheral visual field defects.

Cortical visual impairment is the leading cause of bilateral blindness in children in the developed world. Many children now survive neonatal brain ischaemia or early childhood brain injury, and both are occasionally associated with visual cortical damage. Because of its epidemiological importance, several studies have investigated the outcome and possible management strategies of this condition. Most children show improvement with time; however, it is rare to recover vision completely. An intensive rehabilitation programme should be implemented to help the child to achieve the best physical, sensory, cognitive and linguistic development.

Adult complete (bilateral) cortical blindness is much less common; it is usually overshadowed by hemi-anopia, secondary to unilateral damage of the visual pathway, which is a common complication of stroke. The incidence of complete cortical blindness is unknown. Common causes are stroke, coronary angiography, neoplasms and traumatic head injury. The most important poor prognostic factor is old age. Almost all affected children will recover some of their vision, but elderly patients do not. It is rare for patients over 40 years of age to show improvement a few weeks after the onset. Extensive bioccipital damage and the association of complete cortical blindness with cognitive, behavioural or communication impairments are also poor prognostic indicators. Associated impairments not only make the disabilities much more complex but also make any trial of therapy and rehabilitation extremely difficult.

Adult patients usually present with a fascinating clinical picture. The anterior part of the visual pathway is usually intact, and this can be demonstrated by a normal ophthalmic examination including intact papillary reflexes. The patient reports no conscious experience to any visual stimuli. However, a number of studies have demonstrated that patients with complete cortical blindness can discriminate between different colours, shapes and objects while they insist that they cannot see the stimuli. It has been suggested that this remaining but non-conscious visual capacity is produced by the extrastriatal cortex by-passing the striatal cortex and involving structures such as the amygdala and posterior thalamus, which are not usually affected in such patients. In **Anton's syndrome**, cortical blindness is accompanied by a denial of blindness. The patient is able to confabulate details about his surroundings that may give the appearance of accurate visual abilities.

A standard visual rehabilitation programme usually takes two different approaches. The first is enhancement of the residual vision and the second is using other sensory mechanisms to compensate for the impaired vision. Optical aids such as magnifying lenses are often used for reading or near vision, and large print can also be tried to facilitate reading. The patient's environment should also be assessed and alterations implemented such as increasing lighting or removing dangerous obstacles that may lead to falls.

A visual rehabilitation programme usually aims at encouraging the use of other senses, for example listening to talking books or using voice recognition software. Similar objects (CDs or cassettes) can be recognised using tactile sense by attaching special stickers. Sense of smell can also be enhanced, especially for leisure activities.

Unfortunately, a patient with cortical blindness plus complex visual, cognitive or communication impairments can find it extremely difficult to cope with a standard visual rehabilitation programme. If a patient has visual hallucination, an *enhancement* of residual vision approach might be contraindicated. Increasing visual stimulation is often associated with worsening of the visual hallucinations and a subsequent increase in the patient's confusion and distress. Enhancing the use of other sensations and environmental modulation are probably more appropriate methods to help the patient. However, modest and realistic goals need to be formulated as a demanding programme may increase the patient's distress and discourage further participation.

Some researchers suggest repetitive visual stimulation as a way to stimulate the cells adjacent to the cortical area of functional loss. Results have been encouraging but more robust evidence will be needed for such an approach to be used in routine clinical practice.

Patients with complete cortical blindness can present with unique problems. Sleep disturbance is very common as the patient loses the visual sense of light and finds it difficult to keep a sleep rhythm. This problem can lead to worsening confusion and occasional aggression. It also makes it difficult to implement a suitable care plan. Managing this problem is usually difficult, especially in the early stages after the onset. Trying to control the environment by avoiding stimulation at night, good sleep hygiene and a structured plan for daily activities are usually helpful. Sedatives should be avoided as they may increase the confusion. Melatonin can be tried in selected patients to regulate the sleep rhythm.

The combination of visual hallucinations and cognitive impairment can be a frightening experience for the patients and some of them become agitated and aggressive. A chart of 'antecedent, behaviour, consequence' can be tried to see if there is any pattern and to try to stop any precipitating factors. Spontaneous aggression can occasionally indicate an occipital or temporal lobe epileptic foci, and further assessment is needed with possibly use of antiepileptic drugs.

In general, the prognosis for complete cortical blindness following a stroke is poor and this should be considered when planning the rehabilitation programme. The rehabilitation team should provide constant advice and support to the patient's family as they are often overwhelmed with the unusual presentation and the potentially very demanding situation they have to cope with.

Further reading

Hamm, A. O., Weike, A. I., Schupp, H. T., et al. (2003). Affective blind sight: intact fear conditioning to a visual cue in a cortically blind patient. *Brain* **126**, 267–275.

Widdig, W., Pleger, B., Rommel, O., et al. (2003). Repetitive visual stimulation: a neuropsychological approach to the treatment of cortical blindness. *Neurorehabilitation* **18**, 227–237.

Visual spatial neglect

A 64-year-old man was transferred to the rehabilitation ward after suffering from a right hemisphere stroke. The CT scan showed evidence of right fronto-parietal lobe infarction. Clinical assessment showed left-sided hemiparesis in conjunction with a significant personal and extra-personal neglect.

Comments

The syndrome of unilateral neglect is defined as a failure to report, orient towards or respond to stimuli on the contralesional side or space that cannot be attributed to sensory or motor dysfunction. The neglect phenomenon can be either personal or extra-personal. In personal neglect, the patient neglect the contralesional side of his/her body, resulting in neglect of shaving or grooming of the affected side or unconcern about the motor or sensory deficits. In extra-personal (spatial) neglect, patients are not aware of objects in their contralateral extra-personal space. Personal and extra-personal neglect usually coexist and many patients have poor insight of the impairment (**anosognosia**).

The exact incidence of spatial neglect after either dominant or non-dominant hemispheric injury is not known. However, neglect following non-dominant hemispheric damage is common, with more than half of the patients developing clinically significant neglect. Neglect following dominant hemisphere damage is rare. The reason for such lateralisation of the neglect phenomenon has intrigued scientists. The non-dominant hemisphere is strongly associated with spatial attention, probably with the ability to maintain spatial attention to both sides of space, while the dominant hemisphere can provide only spatial attention to the contralateral (usually right) side. According to this hypothesis, no spatial deficit will result from damage to the dominant hemisphere, as the non-dominant hemisphere will be able to cover the right and left spatial space/body. Non-dominant hemisphere damage, however, will lead to a loss of the contralateral spatial attention function while the intact dominant lobe will be able to maintain spatial attention to its contralateral domain.

Patients with either homonymous hemianopia or spatial neglect will show evidence of a visual field defect affecting the contralateral side. Differentiation between the two conditions is important as rehabilitation, prognosis and even medicolegal aspects can differ, for example, patients with visual field defects can occasionally be allowed to drive or use an outdoor powered wheelchair if they can demonstrate an ability to compensate for their impairment by scanning, but patients with spatial neglect will find it extremely difficult to implement the same methods and drive safely.

Clinical assessment of spatial neglect usually relies on pen and paper tests, such as cancellation, line bisection, or drawing tasks (Table 14.1). These tests fail to consider the patients' actual performances in their everyday lives, with some patients managing to obtain a normal performance rating on conventional tests while suffering from considerable difficulties in daily life skills. Such dissociations have been attributed to the relative sparing of voluntary orientation of attention (involved in conventional tests) contrasting with an impairment of automatic orientation, which allows

Table 14.1. Clinical tests for assessment of neglect

Test	Description
Star cancellation test	A standard test for neglect; the patient is given a piece of paper covered by small letters and stars and is asked to cancel only the stars
Line bisection	Patient tries to mark the halfway point in a number of lines of different lengths
Copying a symmetrical drawing	For example a clock-face
Catherine Bergagego test	A behavioural test in which the patient completes a questionnaire asking about activities that are usually affected by neglect, e.g. shaving or dressing

attention to be automatically captured by relevant stimuli in everyday life. Therefore, evaluation of the impact of spatial neglect on activities of daily living should be considered as an essential element of the assessment process.

Unilateral spatial neglect has consistently been identified as a negative predictor for a patient's recovery. This fact made spatial neglect a prime target for specific pharmacological or therapeutic interventions aiming at reducing its severity and improving the patient's attentional function directed to the specific area of neglect. A key element that should be considered when evaluating these interventions is to determine which techniques achieved improvement in the severity of neglect that was *generalised* and *sustained* for everyday activities outside of the training environment.

The use of catecholamines, particularly methylphenidate, for attentional deficits is well established. Animal studies have suggested that deficiency of the transmitter dopamine is implicated in the pathogenesis of spatial neglect. This observation inspired several studies using dopamine agonists for treatment, with bromocriptine the drug most commonly used. It is extremely difficult to interpret the results of such small trials because of their methodological deficiencies and mixed results. A reasonable approach is to consider bromocriptine for patients with spatial neglect that is associated with a more generalised attentional impairment including significant difficulties resulting from apathy and lack of motivation.

Several therapeutic strategies have been evaluated for the management of spatial neglect. **Scanning training** is a well-known approach to treat patients with pure visual field defects, and evidence is available to support its use with spatial neglect as well. Visual scanning can reduce neglect within a particular task (e.g. in reading by cueing patients to find a red line marked on the left margin). Unfortunately, patients demonstrated little generalisation of their improved scanning behaviour to tasks outside of the training environment.

Prism adaptation, using lenses that induce a rightward horizontal displacement of visual fields is a promising technique. Recent studies have suggested that it may result in long-lasting improvement of neglect that generalises across a wide range of deficits and activities.

Another intervention that has caused considerable excitement recently is **neck muscle vibration**. Vibration of the contralesional neck muscles have produced lasting and more efficient reduction of neglect symptoms than can be obtained by standard treatments. Neck muscle vibration can be carried out in parallel with other treatments and requires low-cost vibration technology, such as that used in physiotherapy. It is well suited for clinical use as an ideal add-on technique in neglect rehabilitation.

Constraint-induced therapy is based on the theory that a patient with a weakness/neglect in a limb will tend to ignore it after time even after sufficient power is regained. Restraining the normal limb with a sling or a mitt will force the patient to use the affected limb. The literature indicates some success of such an approach in patients with hemiparesis. The results in patients with personal neglect were inconclusive. The same approach has been implemented in the management of patients with spatial neglect by using eye patches to block vision in the normal visual field. Again the results of such an approach were mixed.

Another approach to reduce spatial neglect is to increase the hemispheric activation supplying the affected space by providing repetitive stimulation to that hemisphere using simple means such as hand movement. This approach can be easily integrated within the therapy sessions and other activities by advising therapists, nurses and visitors to approach the patient from the affected side and talk or do his personal care from this side.

Further reading

Parton, A., Husain, M. (2004). Spatial neglect. *Adv Clin Neurosci Rehabil* **4**, 18–19.

Samuel, R. P., Buxbaum, L. J. (2002). Treatment of unilateral neglect: a review. *Arch Phys Med Rehabil* **83**, 256–268.

Schindler, I., Kerkhoff, G., Karnath, H.-O. (2002). Neck muscle vibration induces lasting recovery in spatial neglect. *J Neurol Neurosurg Psychiatry* **73**, 412–419.

15

Prescriptions for independence

One of the most interesting aspects of medical rehabilitation practice is the physician's ability to assess several issues and problems facing their patients, such as their seating, posture, gait, cognitive function, etc. These skills enable the treating physician to prescribe non-pharmacological interventions such as exercise or mobility aids. The physician can also formulate management plans involving other therapists or agencies confidently. The physician's knowledge about the different interventions such as vocational rehabilitation or driving assessment puts him/her in a privileged position, as he/she is able to counsel the patient and liase directly with other services with minimal risk of inappropriate referrals or wasting of a rehabilitation potential for the patient.

Exercise prescription

A 62-year-old man recovered very well from a left hemisphere stroke. The residual impairments were mild right hemiparesis with mild gait impairment caused by a combination of weakness, spasticity and poor balance. The patient had a history of hypertension and cardiovascular disease. He has admitted that he was very unfit before his stroke and he is keen to follow a regular exercise programme.

Comments

The aim of most exercise programmes is to increase the physiological capacity of the energy systems most important for a specific activity. The energy needed for muscular activities could be derived from either anaerobic or aerobic pathways (Table 15.1). Anaerobic mechanisms provide high energy

Table 15.1. Main pathways for energy generation

Mechanism of energy production	ATP–creatine phosphate	Anaerobic glycolysis	Aerobic metabolism
Need for oxygen	None	None	Yes
Substrate	High-energy phosphate bonds	Carbohydrates	Carbohydrates, fats or proteins
Metabolism	Breakdown of ATP to ADP and energy	Lactic acid release limits long-term value	Tricarboxylic acid cycle and oxidative phosphorylation; produces CO_2, H_2O and energy
Duration of action	Immediate but limited to 30 seconds	Immediate but limited to few minutes	Unlimited
Activities	Sprinting	Sprinting	Walking, swimming
Exercises	Strengthening, flexibility, balance	Strengthening, flexibility, balance	Aerobic exercise

ATP, adenosine triphosphate; ADP, adenosine disphosphate.

independent of oxygen supply. The reserves to support these mechanisms are very limited and can only be maintained for a few minutes; consequently these mechanisms support short, intense activity such as sprinting or weight lifting. The aerobic pathway, by comparison, provides an unlimited supply of energy and is essential for most daily or sporting activities such as walking, jogging or swimming.

Regular aerobic exercise is needed to maintain health and well-being for any healthy individual. The standard advice is to exercise for at least 30–40 minutes most days of the weeks. The exercise must stretch the cardiovascular system, and a simple way to guide patients is to tell them that they should not be able to speak easily while they are doing the exercise (walking, jogging). Such programmes will have significant health benefits (Table 15.2). It is important to emphasise the benefits of maintaining the exercise programme regularly. Increasing the intensity or duration of the exercise before or afterwards cannot compensate for skipping a week or two without exercise.

Intensity, duration and *frequency* are the three essential components of an exercise prescription. For an aerobic exercise programme, the intensity is usually determined by first establishing the maximal heart rate, which is measured during a symptom-limited exercise stress test. The exercise intensity recommended is usually 60–90% of this rate. Considerations of the

Table 15.2. Health benefits from regular exercise

Reduction of cardiovascular disease risk
Maintenance of bone density
Reduction of lipid levels
Weight reduction
Blood pressure regulation
Reduction of risk of type 2 diabetes mellitus
Improvement in sleep
Reduction in cancer risk
Reduction of overall mortality
Improvement of quality of life

---

patient's age, current level of fitness, presence of a comorbidity such as cardiovascular, respiratory or a neurological disorder will influence the intensity of exercise. The duration of the exercise should be at least 20 minutes and it should be carried out at least three times a week. The exercise should be continuous and rhythmic, using the large muscle groups of the body. The aerobic capacity of the individual can be monitored using the measurement of VO_2 max, which is defined as the maximal amount of oxygen that an individual can consume and use during exercise or physical work. It is measured by analysing the expired air while an individual is performing a maximal exercise test.

Improving individual aerobic capacity will have several beneficial effects. The most significant is the improvement in the heart stroke volume, which is independent of the increase in heart rate. Paradoxically, the individual's resting heart rate falls as his aerobic capacity improves. The improvement in stroke volume is believed to be a result of increasing preload and myocardial contractility.

Strengthening, flexibility and *balance* are the other exercises usually prescribed for individual patients. These exercises are mainly dependent on the anaerobic pathways and they can aim at different adaptations to the exercised muscle groups, such as increasing muscle mass, muscle fibre conversion or adaptations to the neural supply of the muscle. Strengthening exercises are not a standard method of exercise in neurological rehabilitation as they are usually used after injury or as part of sports medicine practice.

Stretching (flexibility) is a common form of exercise recommended for patients with neurological impairments. The exercise programme aims at improving or maintaining the ability to move the joints of the body through their maximal range of movement. Different techniques can be used such as static stretching and static stretching with contraction of the antagonist or agonist muscles. Static stretching is done by slowly moving the joint to the end of its range of movement and then holding it for a period up to a minute, Static stretching with contraction of the antagonist muscle aims at reducing the effects of the stretch reflex, while static stretching with contraction of the agonist muscle aims at providing additional stretch on the connective tissue surrounding the joint, thus achieving greater range of movement. The flexibility exercises should be repeated three to five times in a session and done daily.

For many elderly patients with recurrent falls, patients with inner ear diseases or patients with mild ataxia, balance (proprioception) exercises are very helpful. For patients with mild problems and low risk, simple exercises can be taught and CDs, books and equipment can be suggested. Patients with more severe problems or at high risk could have physiotherapy supervision for their exercises.

Further reading

American College of Sports Medicine (1995). *Guidelines for Exercise Testing and Prescription.* Baltimore, MD: Williams & Wilkins.

Duncan, G. E., Anton, S. D., Sydeman, S. J. (2005). Prescribing exercise at varied levels of intensity and frequency: a randomised trial. *Arch Intern Med* **165**, 2362–2369.

Myslinski, M. J. (2005). Evidence-based exercise prescription for individuals with spinal cord injury. *J Neurol Phys Ther* **29**, 104–106.

Vocational rehabilitation

A 28-year-old man sustained a moderately severe head injury following a road traffic accident. He made a full physical recovery but formal neuropsychological assessment revealed mild attention, memory and high executive function impairment. The patient was married with two children and used to work as a financial adviser. He seeks the support of the rehabilitation team to get back to employment.

Comments

Return to full-time employment is usually considered as the 'icing on the cake', of any successful rehabilitation programme for brain injury. Obvious benefits of employment such as financial independence and full integration into society are extremely important. However, more subtle benefits such as restoration of self-esteem and confidence are probably as important but more difficult to measure.

Table 15.3. Good prognostic factors for return to work

Young age
High level of education
Minimal physical and cognitive disability
Skilled, professional high status employment pre-injury
Married male

Clinicians often concentrate on the severity of the patient's physical and cognitive disabilities as the main prognostic indicators of vocational rehabilitation. Published studies, however, have failed to confirm such a close relationship between the classic biomedical outcomes of brain injury and the possibility of returning to work. Paradoxically, psychosocial premorbid factors such as age, alcohol and drug misuse, status and type of work before injury, and level of education seem to be the most influential factors determining the patient's prognosis from a vocational standpoint. Appreciation of this fact is crucial, as reliance on the biomedical outcomes may lead to a flawed stratification process, with inappropriate patients accessing limited vocational rehabilitation resources while other patients with better prognosis are excluded (Table 15.3).

The poor prognosis for vocational rehabilitation for unskilled and semiskilled workers, despite having minimal physical or cognitive impairments, is difficult to explain. One theory is that brain injury often leads to subtle motor and coordination impairments that are difficult to assess in routine neurological examination. Such impairments may result in significant difficulties in performing a manual job. Satisfaction with a poorly paid and non-stimulating job may also be limited, affecting the patient's motivation to be involved in the rehabilitation programme. A professional person may be more motivated and may also be able to rely on a wide circle of support and colleagues to whom some work can be delegated in the early stages of returning to work.

Again, concentrating on the biomedical issues during a vocational rehabilitation programme might not be the easiest way to achieve a successful outcome. Cognitive rehabilitation programmes can usually lead to modest improvement but trying to influence environmental and psychosocial barriers can also achieve significant goals; for example, ensuring transportation to the work place or installing particular equipment in the work place can dramatically improve the patient's prospects.

Vocational rehabilitation should commence at the acute stage. Patients in employment will find it much easier to return to their original job than to find a new one. Negotiations with the employer should start immediately to try to ensure the patient's rights. In some cases, this approach is clearly inappropriate, as the nature of the job will make it extremely unlikely for the patient to return with his/her physical impairments. Negotiating a fair settlement would be a more suitable approach in such cases.

For most patients, the rehabilitation team should be able to ease them back to employment. Occupational therapists and psychologists are usually in the forefront and a close relationship with occupational health professionals can usually smooth out any issues. Getting back to work part time and with fewer responsibilities are standard recommendations as they help the supporting team to identify any issues early on and tackle them accordingly.

Formal vocational rehabilitation programmes will be needed for many patients. The practice models and the service-delivery methods vary greatly, as do the ways to ensure funding for such programmes. Formal vocational rehabilitation programmes usually accept patients with good potential for rehabilitation. One of the usual exclusion criteria is progressive neurological conditions such as multiple sclerosis or Parkinson' s disease. All vocational rehabilitation programmes encompass two basic concepts: vocational guidance and counselling followed by on-the-job training.

The period of guidance and counselling usually lasts for weeks to months according to the service model and the severity of the patient's condition. Some programmes are residential as they integrate real-life skills and activities of daily living with vocational rehabilitation activities. The programme usually encourages the patient to explore various vocational activities and tries to help in setting realistic expectations about work. The programme also helps the patient to develop skills in areas such as writing a curriculum vitae and interviewing techniques.

On-site development of job skills is usually supported by a **job coach** and it can take place either in an environment simulating a work environment or in the real job environment once employment is secured. The concept of a job coach has revolutionised the practice of vocational rehabilitation as the job coach's responsibilities extend from working with the patient in the work environment to other ways to support and advice the patient about other relevant issues such as financial concerns.

Supported employment is another option to assist patients with disabilities to secure and maintain employment. The employee usually works in an integrated setting with other non-disabled workers, with provision of the supported work maintained by multi-agency funding. The work is paid and the cost effectiveness of the programme is calculated by comparing the programme costs with the worker's earnings.

Further reading

Keyser-Marcus, C. A., Bricout, J. C., Wehman, P. (2002). Acute predictors of return to employment after traumatic brain injury: a longitudinal follow up. *Arch Phys Med Rehabil* **83**, 635–641.

Wehman, P., Kregol, J., Keyser-Marcus, C. A. (2003). Supported employment for persons with traumatic brain injury: a preliminary investigation of long term follow up costs and programme efficiency. *Arch Phys Med Rehabil* **84**, 192–196.

Driving assessment

A 56-year-old man with moderate residual deficits from a left-hemisphere stroke that occurred two years ago attended the mobility centre for advice and an assessment regarding the adaptations required to enable him to drive. He had no visual–perceptual deficits but had severe right-sided weakness of both upper and lower limbs, decreased fine motor skills in the right hand, and problems with balance, especially when fatigued.

Comments

The use of a private motor vehicle has become an essential part of everyday life. Driving frequently serves as the key to independence and is often viewed as a barometer of normality. The performance of domestic tasks, working and involvement in leisure activities are heavily reliant on an individual's ability to drive.

During a medical consultation, patients with clear contraindications to drive because of conditions such as seizures or dense visual field defects can be easily identified. It is extremely difficult to advise other patients with significant cognitive impairments or physical disability about their ability to drive. Such patients often need a formal evaluation by a specialist driving-assessment service.

The assessment procedure can be broadly divided into two components: the pre-drive component of the assessment and the in-car evaluation. Following the confirmation of the client's personal and medical details, the assessment initially focuses upon the physical condition. This is intended to ascertain the level of impairment and determine the client's functional abilities relating to the operation of vehicle controls; it includes measurement of limb strength, range of movement and tolerance to exercise.

Specific cognitive and perceptual tests are not routinely used in the assessment process where there is no question of the client's capacity, as their usefulness remains the subject of much debate. Most agree, however, that although these tests may assist in identifying an area of concern they are unable to provide a clinically reliable means of assessing fitness to drive.

As part of this physical assessment, testing of visual acuity and peripheral vision is made. Clients are required to read a vehicle number plate at a distance of 20 metres. They are also required to have peripheral vision of 120 degrees in the horizontal plane.

On successful completion of the visual requirements, the client is then tested using the mobility centre's static assessment rig. This testing facility comprises a simulated vehicle cockpit that is linked to an onboard computer measuring system.

The current model of static assessment rig in use in the United Kingdom mobility centres was designed to be a multi-test driver assessment facility with interchangeable driving controls, to allow people of varying physical ability to be tested. The unit enables assessors to conduct preliminary tests of the client's use of vehicle controls without using an actual vehicle. Accurate measurements of torque, force, reaction times, decision making and field of vision can be recorded using the battery of tests. Measurements of ergonomic needs are also possible using the static assessment rig.

The selection of the vehicle and vehicle modifications for the in-car assessment is based on the findings of the pre-driving assessment. In the case of someone with a dense right hemiplegia, this is likely to be a vehicle fitted with automatic transmission, power-assisted steering, a left foot accelerator system, a steering spinner and a remote keypad system. An automatic transmission vehicle negates the need to use the left leg to operate the clutch pedal and the left arm for gear selection. Power-assisted steering is always useful for an individual steering with only one arm as it reduces the effort required. The remote keypad is usually combined with a steering wheel spinner. The combined unit is situated on the left side of the steering wheel in a position to suit and allows simultaneous operation of the wheel and secondary controls such as indicators, horn, windscreen wipers and lights. The left foot accelerator pedal is situated to the left of the standard foot brake. A system that ensures there is only one accelerator pedal in position at any one time is the safest option, as this reduces the risk of pressing the accelerator pedal that is not in use at the time by mistake. A twin flip system is used at the time of assessment. This system also allows the accelerators to be changed easily for other people to drive the vehicle.

It is necessary in the first instance to familiarise an individual with the new method of driving. This is done in a private and enclosed area. The vehicle used is also fitted with an instructor's brake. Seating and posture is also addressed and additional lateral support is provided if sitting balance is an issue. The client undertakes manoeuvres under instruction. These involve moving off and stopping under control. Initially, braking can be quite harsh and may need practise to develop sensitivity in the left foot. Manoeuvres are then undertaken to investigate car control and spatial skills. These are all carried out initially without the use of the keypad. The keypad would then be introduced and used to operate the indicators for change in direction.

Use of unfamiliar modifications can complicate the evaluation of someone's driving ability. For example, the concentration required when learning to use the left foot accelerator pedal could demand increased attention, as could using the remote keypad, particularly if being operated by the nondominant hand. A common observation when someone is driving with a remote keypad for the first time is that they often need to attend to the control visually, which can result in a temporary lack of steering control. With the left foot accelerator pedal, it is not uncommon for someone to press the accelerator instead of the brake, particularly if past experience has been with driving using the left foot for operation of a clutch pedal. For all these reasons, it is recommended that a course of professional tuition in a suitably adapted vehicle is undertaken before driving unaccompanied.

To ensure there are no residual cognitive or perceptual symptoms impacting on driving ability, a full on-road assessment can be undertaken once the individual is familiar with the modified driving technique. This involves a comprehensive drive in a range of road and traffic situations to address areas such as decision making and road position.

Further reading

Mazer, B. L., Korner-Bitensky, N. A., Sofer, S. (1998). Predicting ability to drive after stroke. *Arch Phys Med Rehabil* **79**, 743–749.

McKenna, P. (1998). Fitness to drive: a neuropsychological perspective. *J Mental Health* **7**, 9–18.

Part III

Exercises in neurological rehabilitation

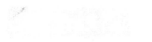

Multiple choice questions

In the following questions, the best single answer should be chosen.

1. A 58-year-old man had a left hemisphere stroke that left him with right-sided weakness and speech problems. On assessment, his speech was fluent but lacked content and included frequent paraphasias. The patient's comprehension seemed intact but his ability to name objects was mildly impaired. The most striking finding was the patient's inability to repeat words or sentences. The most probable diagnosis of this communication impairment is:

    A. Wernicke's aphasia
    B. Conduction aphasia
    C. Sensory trans cortical aphasia
    D. Motor trans cortical aphasia
    E. Broca's aphasia

2. In a routine biochemical and haematological testing, a patient with post-traumatic epilepsy was found to have impaired liver function tests with alanine aminotransferase of 675 U/l and aspartate aminotransferase of 423 U/l. The serum levels of proteins, billirubin and alkaline phosphatase were all within normal range. Full blood count, bone profile, urea and electrolytes were also normal. Which of the drugs the patient is taking is the most probable cause of this biochemical abnormality:

    A. Baclofen
    B. Ibuprofen
    C. Lamotrigine
    D. Sodium valproate
    E. Clobazam

3. A 48-year-old man was admitted to the rehabilitation unit following a closed head injury four days previous. The patient had a fall at home and was found at the bottom of the stairs. Computed tomography showed small left subdural haematoma in conjunction with evidence of mild generalised atrophic changes. The patient had a history of excessive alcohol abuse. On admission to the rehabilitation unit, the patient was disorientated and confused. He exhibited aggressive and violent behaviour and the staff found it difficult to cope with him. The most appropriate drug management at this stage is:

A. Haloperidol
B. Carbamazepine and propranolol
C. Phenytoin
D. Chlordiazepoxide and thiamine
E. Amantadine

4. A 46-year-old woman had a 23-year history of primary progressive multiple sclerosis. In the previous two years, her symptoms deteriorated and she started to use two crutches for outdoors mobility. Clinically, she had evidence of spastic paraplegia and mild ataxia with the right side more severely affected. The patient gave a three-month history of increasing upper limb pain, which was more severe at night. The pain was more severe in the right side and affected mainly the hands and the forearms. Neurological examination of the arms showed normal motor power and sensation in the upper limbs with mild ataxia, which was more severe in the right side. The patient was taking no regular medications. The pain is most probably caused by:

A. Central (thalamic) pain
B. Neuralgic amyotrophy
C. Peripheral neuropathy
D. Radiculopathy
E. Carpal tunnel syndrome

5. A 23-year-old man was admitted for rehabilitation following a severe closed head injury. The patient progressed very well with his rehabilitation and started to mobilise around the ward independently four months following the onset. The patient was pleased he had lost about two stones (around 12.7 kg) following the injury as he had been overweight before the accident. During the ward round, the patient reported a 'funny' sensation in his right thigh, which had started few weeks previously. Clinically, the patient had evidence of mild spastic weakness in his lower limbs, as evident by mild pyramidal weakness and brisk tendon reflexes. There was a band of sensory changes in the lateral aspect of his

right thigh, which was not documented on his admission clerking. The diagnosis is:

A. Lumbar radiculopathy
B. Meralgia paraesthetica
C. Central sensory loss
D. Femoral neuropathy
E. Sciatica

6. A 27-year-old man was admitted to the rehabilitation unit following a severe traumatic brain injury. The patient had several facial injuries including loss of most of his front teeth. Five months after the injury, the patient continued to have significant problems with his swallowing and speech. He was very distressed with the excessive salivation and drooling, which made him embarrassed as he was almost constantly trying to wipe his saliva. All these measures are appropriate at this stage except:

A. Referral for dental management
B. Botulinum toxin injection of the parotid glands
C. Irradiation of the parotid glands
D. Hyoscine patches
E. Oral anticholinergic drugs

7. A 34-year-old man made an excellent recovery from Guillain–Barré syndrome. In his clinic review six months after the onset, clinical examination showed evidence of right foot drop, which in conjunction with sensory and proprioception impairment in the same foot affected his gait. The patient reported a few falls and was keen to improve the quality of his gait. All these measures could be considered except:

A. Walking aids
B. Physiotherapy
C. Raising the heels of his shoes
D. An ankle – foot orthosis
E. Functional electrical stimulation

8. A 58-year-old man had a massive posterior stroke that led to severe cortical blindness and complex cognitive and behavioural problems. One of the behavioural problems that his wife found most distressing was his impulsive need to stand up every few seconds when sitting. This symptom made it extremely difficult for her to take her husband out, as he was unable to tolerate sitting in the car or anywhere without having

this urge to move. The diagnosis was akathesia. The drug of first choice for this condition is:

A. Propranolol
B. Carbamazepine
C. Sodium valproate
D. Clonazepam
E. Haloperidol

9. A 19-year-old man with severe cerebral palsy and lower limb spasticity has tried several combinations of oral antispasticity drugs and botulinum toxin injections with minimal benefit. Two options were discussed with the patient, intrathecal baclofen or intrathecal phenol injections. The following are advantages of intrathecal baclofen over intrathecal phenol except:

A. Reversible
B. More potent
C. No sensory complications
D. Does not affect continence
E. Lower risk of pressure sores in the long term

10. A 19-year-old man was admitted to hospital following a road traffic accident. In the accident and emergency department, the patient assumed a decorticate posture with his shoulders flexed and adducted. The patient responded to pain by opening his eyes and his arms attempted to remove the painful stimulus (supraorbital pressure). The patient could not respond to simple commands and his verbal responses were incomprehensible moans and groans with no clear words spoken and no eye opening. The patient's Glasgow Coma Score is:

A. 6
B. 7
C. 8
D. 9
E. 10

11. Two months after onset, a patient with a C4 complete spinal injury asked about the probable functional outcome for the injury. In the future, this patient should be able to:

A. Eat independently using an aid
B. Help in dressing the upper half of the body
C. Transfer across level surfaces with help
D. Operate an environmental control system
E. Drive an adapted car using hand straps

12. A 64-year-old man who was severely disabled by end-stage multiple sclerosis complained of a problem with sleep rhythm. The patient was up all night and asleep most of the day. His family had tried different ways to reverse his sleep rhythm, such as opening windows during the day and getting him out in the garden, but the patient continued to have this problem. You may like to suggest:

A. Modafinil
B. Amantadine
C. Melatonin
D. Amitriptyline
E. Temazepam

13. A 34-year-old man with dystrophia myotonica has several problems because of the severity of his myotonia. He mentioned dysarthria and hand function as specific problems and enquired if anything could be done to help. The first recommendation should be:

A. Regular stretching exercise
B. Regular strengthening exercise
C. 'Warming-up' technique
D. Phenytoin
E. Neostigmine

14. A 46-year-old man presented to the rehabilitation clinic with worsening memory problems. He had a closed head injury eight years ago from which he made an excellent recovery and was only left with mild short-term memory impairment. The patient managed to hold a full-time job as a guard but was made redundant six months ago. The patient admitted that his memory had been stable for the last eight years since the accident and that he noticed the deterioration only a few months before. The most probable cause of the complaint is:

A. Depression
B. Brain atrophy
C. Early dementia
D. Recent head injury
E. Small vessel disease

15. A 78-year-old woman with a 15-year history of Parkinson's disease presented with significant deterioration of the control of her disease. She complained of frequent *off* periods and found that she had to use

small doses of levodopa every few hours. The following medications may help the patient, apart from:

A. Apomorphine
B. Dopamine agonists
C. Catecholamine O-methyltransferase (COMT) inhibitors
D. Rivastigmine
E. Selegiline

16. A patient presented with a severe high dysexecutive function syndrome following a head injury. His main difficulties were impulsivity, disinhibition and rigidity of thought. The patient had no insight of his difficulties. He was living with his wife and two teenage daughters. The best early approach to this situation is:

A. Drug management
B. Cognitive rehabilitation
C. Advice and support for family
D. Inpatient rehabilitation
E. Long-term residential placement

17. A 23-year-old woman with spina bifida had a ventriculo-peritoneal shunt inserted after birth to manage hydrocephalus. In the last five years, the shunt has needed to be revised twice. The patient was admitted with a two week history of cognitive deterioration. The patient refused to have a scan to assess her shunt. The patient's capacity to refuse management needed to be determined. The most crucial determinant for capacity is:

A. Accurate cognitive assessment using appropriate psychometric tests
B. The patient's ability to choose rational decisions
C. The severity of the medical condition
D. The patient's ability to understand the procedure and its potential benefits and risks if not performed
E. The patient's ability to speak clearly

18. A 43-year-old man was admitted to the rehabilitation unit after being diagnosed with Guillain–Barré syndrome five days previously. The patient had evidence of ascending neuropathy. Two days after the admission, the patient started to complaint of difficulty talking, swallowing and shortness of breath. The patient was urgently transferred to the intensive care unit where he was artificially ventilated after his blood gases showed:

A. Low oxygen, low carbon dioxide and low pH
B. Low oxygen, high carbon dioxide and high pH

C. Low oxygen, low carbon dioxide and high pH
D. Low oxygen, high carbon dioxide and low pH
E. Low oxygen, normal carbon dioxide, normal pH

19. A 54-year-old woman has had multiple sclerosis for 20 years. She presented to the rehabilitation clinic with lower limb pain over the previous eight months. The patient described the pain as severe, a dull ache in character and affecting mainly the lower limbs. The pain was more severe at rest in the daytime and was almost constant at night. This had led to significant difficulty in getting adequate sleep, with a subsequent daytime fatigue. The patient described an urge to move her feet when the pain was intense. Clinically, the patient's gait was slightly ataxic, but motor power and sensation were normal in the lower limbs. The knee and ankle reflexes were brisk in both limbs and the planters equivocal in the right side and up-going in the left. The most probable cause of pain is:

A. Painful spasms
B. Spino thalamic pain
C. Peripheral neuropathy
D. Ischaemic pain
E. Restless leg syndrome

20. An 83-year-old man had a cerebrovascular stroke four years ago that left him with mild right-sided weakness. The patient also had a 20-year history of hypertension. The patient presented to the rehabilitation clinic having experienced visual hallucinations over the previous six months. The patient and his family described recurrent episodes when he reported seeing several images from his childhood and from the time when he was in the army. Examination of the eyes showed no abnormality. The most probable cause of these hallucinations is:

A. Temporal seizures
B. Psychosis
C. Posterior cortical infarcts
D. Hypertensive encephalopathy
E. Migraine

21. A 21-year-old man presented to the rehabilitation clinic with a diagnosis of Becker's muscle dystrophy. The condition was diagnosed when the patient was 12 years old. He used callipers to mobilise for short distances but relied on a lightweight wheelchair for outdoor

mobility. The patient had several questions about his condition. Which of the following statements is true:

A. Risk of cardiac involvement is minimal
B. The patient's offspring will have a 50% chance of developing the condition
C. The patient should expect a normal life expectancy
D. Urinary incontinence is a recognised feature of the disease
E. Osteoporosis is a recognised late complication

22. A 48-year-old man had developed a cauda equina syndrome secondary to an S1–S2 disc prolapse. The patient presented with bilateral asymmetrical lower limb weakness associated with patchy sensory loss. The patient had difficulty passing urine because of what he described as lack of sensation. His post-micturition volume was 350 ml. Suitable management for his bladder impairment at this stage is:

A. Oral anticholinergic drugs
B. Intermittent self-catheterisation
C. Suprapubic catheter
D. Botulinum toxin injection
E. Condom drainage

23. A 43-year-old woman was diagnosed with multiple sclerosis 12 years ago and presented to the rehabilitation clinic with a five day history of vertigo. The patient suffered from cerebellar ataxia. The following suggest a peripheral cause of the vertigo, except:

A. Severe imbalance
B. Nausea and vomiting
C. Sudden onset
D. Worsening of vertigo with change of position
E. Intermittent

24. A 17-year-old man with mitochondrial myopathy had generalised muscle wasting and weakness in both lower limbs. Bilateral quadriceps muscle wasting and weakness was, however, the outstanding clinical abnormality. The patient hyperextended his knee with his hand when taking weight on it to prevent it buckling beneath him. The patient also had bilateral shortening of his Achilles tendons with restriction of the range of movement of the ankles and limited dorsiflexion. The patient's orthopaedic surgeon suggested lengthening of the Achilles tendons to improve the gait pattern and prevent fixed ankle deformities. The

operation may cause significant deterioration of the patient's gait because:

A. Improvement of dorsiflexion will promote knee flexion
B. Improvement of dorsiflexion will promote knee extension
C. The ground reaction force will move anteriorly
D. Achilles tendon lengthening will destabilise the ankle joint
E. Postoperative complications are common

25. A 23-year-old man with a complete thoracic spinal injury developed headache, flushing and sweating as he was catheterised. A blood pressure of 210/140 mm Hg was rapidly controlled by appropriate antihypertensive drugs. Diagnosis of autonomic dysreflexia was suspected. This disorder is only seen in spinal injuries with a level above:

A. T6
B. T7
C. T8
D. T9
E. T10

26. A 64-year-old woman had a stroke eight years ago that left her with right-sided hemiparesis. Significant spasticity affecting her elbow flexors caused pain and increased the risk of flexion deformity of the right elbow joint. The patient had been receiving botulinum toxin injections to her right biceps and brachioradialis muscles for the last seven years. In the last year, the patient noticed that the injections had become less effective, with increasing pain and difficulty maintaining the stretching of the injected muscles. Secondary unresponsiveness to botulinum toxin was suggested. The next step should be:

A. Consider plasma exchange
B. Consider intravenous immunoglobulin
C. Short course of oral steroids before the next injection
D. Use a different sero type of botulinum toxin
E. Suspend injections for 12 months

27. A 34-year-old man was diagnosed as positive for human immuno-deficiency virus (HIV) in a routine test. The patient was completely asymptomatic and he thought that he must have acquired the infection a few years previously during a casual unprotected sexual contact. For the last two years, the patient had been in a steady relationship and living with a partner in a house that they had jointly

bought. However, his partner decided to leave him and they agreed to sell the house. The patient has found it very difficult to find suitable accommodation and has had to go back to live with his parents; this has led to a 50 mile round trip to drive to work. The patient has:

A. A pathology, impairment, disability and handicap
B. A pathology but no impairment, disability or handicap
C. A pathology, impairment but no disability or handicap
D. A pathology, disability but no impairment or handicap
E. A pathology, handicap but no impairment or disability

28. A 48-year-old man had been diagnosed with multiple sclerosis four years ago but was mobile and only complained of mild spastic paraparesis. In the last six months, the patient had started to complain of diarrhoea, stomach upset, impotence and palpitations. He also complained of severe giddiness when standing. This symptom was caused by a postural reduction in blood pressure. Autonomic neuropathy was suspected as a cause of the symptoms. As autonomic neuropathy is extremely rare in multiple sclerosis, the following conditions need to be excluded except:

A. Diabetes mellitus
B. Amyloidosis
C. Lead poisoning
D. Alcoholic neuropathy
E. Multi system atrophy

29. A 56-year-old man was admitted to hospital with pneumonia. He has had multiple sclerosis for 18 years, which has left him with limited mobility. The patient has had long-term problems with his swallowing and was on a soft diet. Aspiration was suspected as the primary cause of his pneumonia. Swallowing assessment after recovery from the pneumonia showed mildly impaired swallowing; however, the patient managed a soft diet with no problems. The following are appropriate actions at this stage except:

A. Enforce advice regarding the consistency of food and posture while eating and more care when the patient is tired
B. Investigations for reflux oesophagitis
C. Referral for a percutaneous endoscopic gastrostomy (PEG)
D. Videofluoroscpy
E. Referral to a nutritionist

30. A 30-year-old man with post-traumatic epilepsy attended the rehabilitation clinic as he was keen to get back to driving. He had a head injury four years previously. He has been taking lamotrigine 250 mg daily. He last had a seizure 18 months previously and only has occasional auras, with a frequency of about one or two a month. The patient is keen to get back to driving, as it is important to improve his job prospects. The most appropriate action is:

A. Agree that he can get back to driving and reduce the dose of lamotrigine
B. Agree that he can get back to driving and continue with the same dose of lamotrigine
C. Should not get back to driving and reduce the dose of lamotrigine
D. Should not get back to driving and continue with the same dose of lamotrigine
E. Should not get back to driving and increase the dose of lamotrigine

31. A 72-year-old man was admitted to hospital for an elective surgery for an abdominal aortic aneurysm. Two days after the operation he developed sudden paralysis of the lower limbs. The clinical findings at this stage will most probably be:

A. Flaccid paralysis of lower limbs with impaired superficial and deep sensation below T4 level
B. Flaccid paralysis of lower limbs with impaired superficial and preserved deep sensation below level T10
C. Flaccid paralysis of lower limbs with impaired deep sensation and preserved superficial sensation below level T6
D. Flaccid paralysis of the lower limbs with preserved superficial and deep sensation
E. Flaccid paralysis with patchy sensory loss in the lower limbs

32. A 62-year-old woman had a stroke two years ago that left her with a left-sided hemiplegia. The patient had a non-functional right hand with a mildly increased muscle tone in the flexor muscle groups. The patient has been using a hand splint for more than six months to prevent joint deformities and asked if the splint is appropriate. The hand splint should maintain the hand in a position of:

A. Slight extension of the wrist, metacarpophalangeal joints (MCP) and intraphalangeal joints (IP)
B. Slight flexion of the wrist, MCPs and IPs
C. Slight extension of the wrist, MCPs and flexion of IPs

D. Slight flexion of the wrist, IPs and flexion of MCPs

E. Slight extension of the wrist, IPs and flexion of MCPs

33. A 23-year-old man has had a severe closed head injury and has been bed bound for two months. At this stage, assessment of his cardiovascular function may reveal:

A. Rest tachycardia

B. Failure to increase heart rate with exercise

C. Increase cardiac output

D. Increase in blood volume

E. Increase peripheral oxygen utilisation

34. A 32-year-old man with a complete spinal injury at T8 presented to the rehabilitation clinic complaining of sexual dysfunction. He has had problems with his libido, penile erection and difficulty maintaining an erection. The following suggestions may help the patient except:

A. Oral sildenafil

B. Vaccum-assisted erection

C. Penile prosthesis

D. Intracavernosal injections

E. Electro-ejaculation

35. A 72-year-old man was diagnosed with motor neurone disease three years ago. In the last four months, his swallowing deteriorated considerably secondary to bulbar muscle involvement. A decision to insert a percutaneous endoscopic gastrostomy (PEG) tube was taken. Two weeks later, the patient continued to have problems with persistent vomiting. At this stage, the following is recommended:

A. Regular antiemetics

B. Change the feeding regimen to continuous instead of bolus feed

C. Upper endoscopy to exclude gastro-oesophageal pathology

D. Discontinuation of PEG feeding for 48 hours

E. Referral to consider jejunostomy

36. A 45-year-old woman was admitted to the rehabilitation unit for the management of a deep sacral pressure sore. The patient was diagnosed with multiple sclerosis 16 years ago and was bed bound for the last two years. The patient was double incontinent and had spastic paraplegia with wind-swept legs. Two weeks after admission, the pressure sore looked much cleaner with almost complete removal of the necrotic

tissue and a healthy hyperaemic floor. Three weeks later, the pressure sore failed to improve further. The following are appropriate measures at this stage except:

A. Maggot therapy
B. Strict bed rest
C. Urethral catheter and regular enemas
D. Negative pressure therapy
E. Plastic surgery consultation

37. A 24-year-old man suffered a closed head injury during a road traffic accident. He made an excellent physical recovery but continued to have significant cognitive problems eight months after the accident. The patient has a wife and a young son and was very keen to participate in a cognitive rehabilitation programme. A formal psychometric assessment showed evidence of impairments in memory, language and high executive function. During consultation, all but one of these approaches were recommended as the standard elements of a cognitive rehabilitation programme; which is not useful?

A. Using residual skills more effectively
B. Avoiding potential problems by restructuring the environment
C. Restoration of the functional aspects of memory
D. Finding different ways to achieve goals
E. Using assistive technology

38. A 38-year-old woman who has had multiple sclerosis for the past 16 years has been wheelchair dependent for the last four years. The patient's main impairments were spastic paraplegia and mild ataxia. The patient used an attendant-propelled wheelchair and sat on a pressure-relieving cushion. Over the last three weeks, the patient's husband has noticed vulnerable areas above her sacrum. Clinically, the patient had a stage 1 sacral pressure sore. The following measure can reduce the pressure over the vulnerable areas:

A. Increase the wheelchair tilt
B. Increase the height of the footrest
C. Lower the backrest
D. Attach a headrest to improve stability
E. Lower the armrest

39. A 21-year-old man had a spinal cord injury following a motorcycle accident. On admission to the hospital, his neurological examination showed a normal sensory and motor level of the C7 myotomes and

dermatomes. Below this level, the patient had complete muscle paralysis but patchy areas of sensation were preserved. The patient also had some preserved sensation in his sacral area. The patient had no anal muscle tone and during examination the anal reflex was not detected. According to the American Spinal Injury Association (ASIA) Impairment Scale, this patient has impairment at level:

A. ASIA A
B. ASIA B
C. ASIA C
D. ASIA D
E. ASIA E

40. A 58-year-old man was reviewed following a cerebrovascular accident four months previously that had left him with right leg weakness. The patient was advised by his physiotherapist to use a walking stick when walking outdoors. The patient felt that the walking stick was not helping his walking and asked if he was using it correctly. The walking stick should:

A. Have a length that extends from the bottom of the heel to a level 20 cm below the hip
B. Be advanced with the ipsilateral leg
C. Have a leather handle
D. Be held in the arm opposite the affected side
E. Painted white

41. A 35-year-old epileptic woman has been well controlled on a daily dose of 200 mg topiramate. She presented with worsening of her epilepsy control with three generalised seizures in the last two months. The patient had started taking complementary and alternative medicine sessions for stress. She noticed that the seizures occurred within 24 hours of having the therapy sessions and was not sure if this was just a coincidence. The most likely cause of this is receiving:

A. Reflexology
B. Homeopathy
C. Indian head massage
D. Acupuncture
E. Aromatherapy

42. A 32-year-old patient with a complete spinal injury at T8 attended the rehabilitation clinic for his annual review. He managed his bladder with intermittent self-catheterisation four times a day. He had a single

urinary tract infection last year and had no incontinence episodes, pain or haematuria in the last year. The most appropriate screening test for this patient is:

A. Abdominal ultrasound
B. A renal radioisotope scan
C. Abdominal plain X-ray
D. Urodynamic studies
E. Assessment of the glomerular filtration rate

43. A 58-year-old man was resuscitated successfully 20 minutes after a cardiac arrest. The patient developed hypoxic brain damage and was managed in intensive care for three weeks. He was transferred to the rehabilitation unit four weeks later. On admission, the patient was confused and disorientated. He suffered from recurrent but brief shock-like jerks of his whole body; however, his right arm and leg seemed to be more affected and their shakes seemed more violent. The jerks were usually spontaneous but seemed also to occur when the patient is touched on particular areas of his body. The drug of first choice to treat this patient is:

A. Haloperidol
B. Propranolol
C. Diazepam
D. Methylphenidate
E. Sodium valproate

44. A 34-year-old female patient was admitted to the rehabilitation unit because of a relapse of her multiple sclerosis. For 10 days, she had noticed considerable worsening of the vision in her right eye in conjunction with double vision. The patient's ataxia and balance seemed also to worsen. The patient received 1 g methylprednisolone intravenously for three days. A two week programme of physiotherapy commenced to improve her gait. Six days after admission, the patient started to complaint to her husband that she was mistreated by the staff and that other patients have been laughing at her. The patient was keen to leave the unit especially because she felt that her therapists were laughing at her as well. The reason for these paranoid delusions is probably:

A. Manic depression
B. Schizophrenic episode
C. Multiple sclerosis relapse
D. Steroids
E. An acute infection

45. A 62-year-old woman was admitted to the rehabilitation unit after suffering from a subarachnoid haemorrhage, which was managed surgically. The patient remained immobile and confused for two weeks following the onset. Hypercalcaemia was detected on routine investigation following the surgery and was thought to result from a combination of immobility and dehydration. As the patient's hypercalcaemia persisted, further investigations were arranged. Results showed a raised corrected calcium level, reduced phosphate level and a high parathyroid hormone assay. The following agents can reduce the calcium level except:

    A. Oral phosphate
    B. Intravenous pamidronate
    C. Calcitonin
    D. Steroids
    E. Furosemide

46. A 68-year-old man was admitted to the rehabilitation unit four days after suffering a stroke that left him with dense right hemiplegia, aphasia and dysphagia. The patient was started on aspirin 325 mg/day for secondary prevention. Six days after admission, the patient had a diarrhoeal episode, which lasted for two days. Three days later, the patient's right calf muscle was noticed to be swollen and deep venous thrombosis was diagnosed using venography. This patient should have:

    A. Started on subcutaneous heparin when the stroke was diagnosed
    B. Used a mechanical device in both limbs to improve venous return
    C. Had a combination of aspirin and clopidogrel for a more robust thromboprophylaxis
    D. Had more aggressive physiotherapy to improve mobility
    E. Been adequately rehydrated during his diarrhoeal illness

47. A 34-year-old man with a spinal injury at C7 attended his annual review in the rehabilitation clinic. He had been keeping in good health since the injury three years ago. During the appointment, clinical examination revealed impaired superficial and pain sensations affecting both hands and the lateral aspect of the forearms. The most appropriate action at this stage is:

    A. Observation and review of the neurological impairments during the following annual review
    B. Nerve conduction studies
    C. Magnetic resonance imaging (MRI) of the wrists
    D. An MRI scan of the cervical spine
    E. A computed tomographic scan of the chest

48. A 48-year-old man was admitted to the rehabilitation unit to improve his mobility. The patient had been critically ill for five months and spent three weeks in the intensive care unit to manage sepsis. The patient's mobility started to improve in the rehabilitation unit but he had significant bilateral foot drop, which seemed to impede his progress. The patient also had significant and fluctuating lower limb oedema, which was difficult to control. Orthotic management can improve the feet drop using:

A. Plastic moulded ankle–foot orthosis (AFO)
B. Double metal upright AFO
C. Patellar tendon bearing AFO
D. A knee–ankle–foot orthosis (KAFO)
E. Heel raise in a surgical shoe

49. A 63-year-old male had suffered a cerebrovascular stroke two years previously that left him with right-sided hemiplegia. He presented to the rehabilitation clinic with right hand pain. Clinically, the patient had increasing muscle tone in the flexor muscles of the wrist and fingers. He also had a thumb-in-hand deformity. It was difficult clinically to extend or abduct the thumb fully and the patient said that it was impossible for him to use his hand splint. To improve the thumb-in-hand deformity, the following muscles should be injected with botulinum toxin:

A. Opponens pollicis, abductor pollicis and lateral two lumbricals
B. Opponens pollicis, adductor pollicis and lateral two lumbricals
C. Opponens pollicis, abductor pollicis and flexor pollicis longus
D. Opponens pollicis, adductor pollicis and flexor pollicis longus
E. Opponens pollicis, lateral two lumbricals and flexor pollicis longus

50. A 59-year-old man has had a four year history of atypical Parkinson's disease. The diagnosis of multisystem atrophy was suggested as the patient suffered from a troublesome autonomic dysfunction and responded poorly to levodopa. The most significant feature of the autonomic dysfunction was a postural fall in blood pressure. The patient had several falls because of this postural problem and was keen to explore any ideas that may help him with this problem. The following measures can help the patient's autonomic dysfunction except:

A. Oral fludrocortisone
B. Oral alpha blockers
C. Oral beta blockers
D. Stockings
E. Avoiding warm weather

Multiple choice answers

1B. Patients with Broca's or motor trans cortical aphasias will present with non-fluent speech. In sensory trans cortical aphasia, the ability to repeat words is maintained. Those with Wernicke's aphasia usually have significant problems with comprehension.

2D. Routine liver function tests are needed for valproate, dantrolene and tizanidine therapy because of the high risk of liver damage.

3D. The scenario suggests delirium tremens secondary to sudden alcohol withdrawal as a contributing cause of the confusion and aggression.

4E. Carpal tunnel syndrome is commonly seen in wheelchair users and also with patients using crutches or walking sticks.

5B. Entrapment of the lateral cutaneous nerve of the thigh (meralgia paraesthetica) is a common complication of sudden weight loss or weight gain. The condition can be bilateral and usually resolves as the patient regains his normal weight. Surgery is rarely needed and is only considered for long-term problems presenting with significant pain.

6C. Dentures, anticholinergic drugs and botulinum toxin injections are standard measures to manage excessive salivation. All these measures are reversible and could be discontinued as the patient improves. Destructive irradiation is irreversible and is usually used in patients with very limited prospects for recovery.

7E. Functional electrical stimulation is contraindicated in peripheral nerve pathology as intact peripheral nerves are needed to transmit the electric stimulus.

8A. Propranolol is the drug of choice for akathesia.

9B. Phenol injections are usually more potent than intrathecal baclofen therapy as phenol completely destroys the nerves involved in the spinal reflexes. The major complications of phenol use are permanent double incontinence and dysthesia.

Table A.1. Glasgow Coma Scale

Item	Response	Score
Eye opening	None	1
	To pain	2
	To speech	3
	Spontaneously	4
Motor response	None	1
	Extension	2
	Abnormal flexion	3
	Withdrawal	4
	Localises pain	5
	Obeys commands	6
Verbal response	None	1
	Incomprehensible	2
	Inappropriate	3
	Confused	4
	Oriented	5

10D. The Glasgow Coma Scale is given in Table A.1.

11D. A patient with a complete C4 lesion will be unable to perform any manual task. However, he will be able to operate an environmental control system using his chin.

12C. Melatonin is very effective in normalising sleep patterns. Modafinil is very useful for isolated daytime somnolence and amantadine for fatigue secondary to multiple sclerosis.

13C. Warming-up techniques include chewing gum before speaking or arm exercise before manual tasks. Contracting the muscles several times before the activity results in faster relaxation and stronger contractions.

14A. Cognitive complications following head injury rarely deteriorate after the post-acute period. Worsening of cognitive function especially attention and memory is usually secondary to a mental health problem such as anxiety or depression.

15D. The main indication for rivastigmine is cognitive and behavioural impairments.

16C. Frontal lobe syndrome following head injury is extremely difficult to manage. The patient's poor insight makes it almost impossible to engage him in any meaningful rehabilitation effort. In severe cases, patients may need to live in a prosthetic environment with minimal disturbance to a fixed daily routine. In milder cases, the patient is often able to continue his community living. The patient's family and carers will need continuing advice and support to learn how to deal with the patient and to cope with the situation.

17D. Assessment of capacity does not aim at determining the patient's general abilities to make judgements. The assessment's main goal is to establish if the patient is able to understand the action proposed, weigh the benefits and risks and communicate a decision. A patient who fulfils these requirements has the capacity to make the decision however irrational it might be. Capacity must be assessed with regard to the situation. On the one hand, a patient with mild cognitive impairment may not have the capacity to manage a complex financial transaction. On the other hand, one with a more severe cognitive impairment may be able to make decisions about where to live or with whom.

18D. The patient will have a type II respiratory failure with hypercapnoea and respiratory acidosis.

19E. The clinical picture is consistent with the diagnosis of restless leg syndrome. This condition is common and can be associated with other neurological conditions. Dopaminergic agonists are the first line of treatment.

20C. Any patient with blindness can develop visual hallucinations whatever the cause of blindness. However, the condition described here is strongly associated with the effects of posterior cortical lacunar infarcts.

21E. Becker's muscle dystrophy is an X-linked recessive genetic disease so sons of the man will not be affected but daughters will be carriers. Cardiac involvement occurs in 50% of patients.

22B. The clinical picture is of a lower motor neurone lesion leading to a flaccid bladder. Intermittent self-catheterisation is the management of choice.

23A. Imbalance and oscillopsia are more severe in cerebellar syndromes. Sudden onset of severe vertigo, which is occasionally associated with nausea and vomiting or cochlear symptoms, is suggestive of a peripheral pathology.

24A. Lengthening of the Achilles tendon will improve the ankle's dorsiflexion; this will subsequently lead to a shifting of the ground reaction force posteriorly, creating a knee flexion moment. Strong quadriceps muscles will be needed to stabilise the knee. Weak quadriceps will be unable to counteract the knee flexion movements, leading to buckling of the knee.

25A. Injuries would be above T6.

26D. All the measures suggested have had some success in the management of antibody formation. However, the standard practice is to switch to another sero type of botulinum toxin.

27E. The patient's pathology is his HIV-positive status. He is asymptomatic, hence has no impairment or disability. However, his handicap is directly secondary to his pathology, having lost his relationship and home. Handicap is not always automatically caused by the disability and disability is also not necessarily caused by the impairment.

28C. Diabetes mellitus, Guillain–Barré syndrome, amyloidosis, alcohol, acute intermittent porphyria and multisystem atrophy can cause autonomic neuropathy.

29C. Non-compliance with the recommendations for safe swallowing is not uncommon. Carers may feel under pressure as the patient is keen to eat his favourite food or is not keen on some recommendations such as fluid thickeners. Advice about posture when the patient is eating and to be extra careful when he is tired or ill is as important as the food consistency recommended. The family or carers can be given a sliding scale of safe foods so they can scale up if the patient is unwell, giving him safer consistencies of food that could be easier to swallow.

30E. Auras are seizures, hence they disqualify the patient from getting back to driving because of the risk of generalisation. As the patient is keen to drive, an effort to eliminate the auras should be made by increasing the dose of his antiepileptic drugs.

31B. More than 60% of cases of spinal stroke are secondary to an abdominal aortic artery pathology. Spinal ischaemia affects mainly the anterior part of the spinal cord supplied by the anterior spinal arteries, thus sparing the dorsal column. The lower thoracic area is the most vulnerable to damage.

32E. Wrist and IPs need slight extension, while the MCPs need flexion.

33A. Rest tachycardia and an exaggerated heart rate response to exercise are extremely common following prolonged immobility. A reduction of the stroke volume leads to reduction in the cardiac output despite the increased heart rate. The reduction in blood volume is caused by the reduced hydrostatic blood pressure in conjunction with a reduction in the secretion of antidiuretic hormone. The cardiovascular changes secondary to prolonged immobility is usually referred to as **cardiovascular adaptation syndrome**.

34E. Electro-ejaculation is only appropriate for fertility treatment and should never be offered to patients as a management option for impotence.

35B. Bolus feeding via the PEG tube is usually more convenient to the patient as it gives a longer period not necessarily attached to the nutritional system. Occasionally, patients fail to tolerate the bolus feeds and a slower rate of feeding is needed. This is usually given throughout the night but care should be taken with the patient's posture to avoid aspiration. Antiemetics, especially if these act to improve gut motility (e.g. meto-cloperamide or domeperidone), may also help. Rarely, jejunostomy will be needed to try to insert the tube in a more distal location.

36A. Maggot therapy is useful in the early stages to remove necrotic tissues and promote hyperaemia. Strict bed rest, appropriate pressure-relieving mattress, improving continence, revision of posture in bed are all appropriate steps at this stage. Early consideration of negative-pressure therapy and surgical intervention may prevent unnecessary delays in healing.

37C. There is no evidence that rehabilitation can restore functional memory.

38A. Increasing the wheelchair tilt will increase the surface area taking the body weight. Lowering the footrest will reduce hip and knee flexion, subsequently increasing the surface area of the thigh in contact with the seat and taking more of the body pressure onto this area. Reducing the height of the back of the seat and lowering the armrests are good strategies to improve the use and function of the upper limbs.

39B. The ASIA classification is the most commonly used measure for accurate description of the neurological impairments following spinal injury (Table A.2).

Table A.2. The American Spinal Injury Association Impairment Scale

ASIA grade	Features
A	Complete; no motor or sensory function is preserved in the sacral segments S2–S4
B	Incomplete; sensory but not motor function preserved below the neurological level including the sacral segments S2–S4
C	Motor function preserved below the neurological level with more than half of the muscles below the lesion at grade 3/5 or less
D	More than half of the muscles below the lesion showing muscle strength greater than 3/5
E	Normal motor and sensory function below the lesion

40D. The most appropriate length for a walking stick is the distance between the bottom of the shoe heel and the ipsilateral greater trochanter. The walking stick should be held in the arm opposite the affected side and should advance with the affected leg.

41E. Some essential oils used in aromatherapy such as rosemary, peppermint and basil have a stimulant effect and can decrease the seizure threshold.

42B. A radioisotope renogram is the most sensitive investigation to pick up any renal damage in an early stage. The test, however, is non-specific. If the renogram is positive, an ultrasound should show any significant structural changes; plain X-ray will detect renal stones and urodynamic studies will provide detailed information about the function of the different parts of the lower renal system, thus indicating the most appropriate method to manage the patient. An impaired glomerular filtration rate is a relatively late manifestation of renal impairment.

43E. The patient has postencephalitic myoclonus. The drug of first choice for management is sodium valproate.

44D. Steroid-induced psychosis is not uncommon. It is usually managed with standard antipsychotic medications. Psychosis is not a recognised feature of multiple sclerosis relapses or acute infections.

45D. The diagnosis is primary hyperparathyroidism. All the drugs mentioned could lower calcium levels except for steroids, which lower high calcium levels secondary to other medical conditions such as sarcoidosis, malignancy or vitamin D overdose. Steroids are not effective in treating hypercalcaemia secondary to primary or tertiary hyperparathyroidism.

46E. Dehydration is one of the low-profile but important precipitating factors for thromboembolism. Neurologically impaired patients are especially vulnerable to even a mild diarrhoeal illness as many of them will have swallowing, communication or cognitive problems, with subsequent difficulty ensuring adequate fluid replacement.

47D. The patient is developing sensory impairments affecting the C6–C7 dermatomes, most probably indicating an extension of the level of the spinal injury upwards. The most probable reason is post-traumatic syringomyelia. An MRI of the cervical spine is the investigation of choice.

48B. Usual types of AFO or KAFO will not be suitable for a patient with massive or fluctuating ankle oedema. A double metal upright AFO uses an unaltered shoe, avoiding any stress on the oedematous feet and ankles. The double metal bars originating from the shoe are connected to a calf band, which is the crucial part stabilising the foot and ensuring a degree of dorsiflexion during the swing phase.

49D. Opponens pollicis and adductor pollicis are injected in the thenar eminence while the flexor pollicis longus muscle is injected in the forearm.

50B. Avoiding sudden change of posture, large meals and warm weather can all help patients with postural blood pressure reduction. Fludrocortisone can improve the symptoms as it increases salt and water retention and beta blockers can help by increasing peripheral vasoconstriction. Alpha blockers, however, will lead to peripheral vasodilatation, with subsequent reduction of the blood pressure.

Index

Note: Page numbers in *italics* refer to tables

Achilles tendon lengthening 113
activity coordinator 7–8
acupuncture 107–8
acute stage
  needs 6
  service provision 6–7
aciclovir 15
Addenbrooke's Cognitive Examination (ACE)
  39
admission of patients 6
adrenocorticotrophic hormone (ACTH) 17,
  18, *19*
aerobic capacity 148
aggression 41–3
  behavioural management 41
  communication strategies 42
  cortical blindness 142
  functional analysis 42
  management 42–3
  pharmacological management 43
  physical restraint 43
  positive feedback 42
agitation
  cortical blindness 142
  herpes simplex encephalitis 15–16
  Huntington's disease 49
  wandering patients 83
agraphia 132
akathesia, Huntington's disease 49
alcohol
  abuse and pontine myelinolysis 35, 36
  seizure trigger 13
allodynia 92
  complex regional pain syndrome 95–6
alpha blockers
  autonomic dysreflexia 27–8
  urine retention with overflow 124–5
alternative medicine *see* complementary and

    alternative medicine
amantadine 34
American Spinal Injury Association (ASIA)
    Impairment Scale 178
amitriptyline 92
amnesia *see* post-traumatic amnesia (PTA)
amputation in Charcot arthropathy 80–1
amyotrophic neuralgia *see* neuralgic amyotrophy
anaemia, pressure sores 65
anal sphincter
  external 128–9
  internal 127
analgesia
  complex regional pain syndrome 96
  neuralgic amyotrophy 120
ankle–foot orthosis (AFO) 80
  equino varus deformity 112
ankle inversion, equino varus deformity 112
anomia 135
anorectal reflex 127
  bowel programme 128
anosognosia 143
antibiotics
  Charcot arthropathy 79–80
  pressure sores 66
antidepressants
  anxiety disorder 22–3
  complex regional pain syndrome 96
  conversion syndrome 103
  herpes simplex encephalitis 16
  see also tricyclic antidepressants
antidiuretic hormone (ADH) 18
antiepileptic drugs 13
  central pain syndrome 92–3
  complex regional pain syndrome 96
  herpes simplex encephalitis 16
  high dosage 14
  wandering patient 84

antipsychotic drugs
  herpes simplex encephalitis 16
  wandering patient 84
antispasticity medications 115
Anton's syndrome 141
anxiety
  following brain injury 20–3
    antidepressants 22–3
    prognosis 23
    symptoms 22
  Huntington's disease 49
apathy
  frontal lobe dysfunction 40
  Huntington's disease 49
aphasia 130–1
  apraxia association 133
  conduction 134–5
  diagnosis 131, 135
  expressive 130–3
  fluent 131–2, 136
  global 131–2
  jargon 134–6
  nominal 131–2
  non-fluent 131–2
  syndromes 131–2
  transcortical 132
applied behaviour analysis 42
apraxia 130–1, 133
  assessment 133
  localization 133
arcuate fasciculus 131
  damage 134–5
arginine stimulation test 18
arm
  function loss after stroke 97–8
  position in hemiplegic painful
    shoulder 99
  TENS 99–100
aromatherapy 108
arteriovenous malformations, cerebral 24
arthrodesis, equino varus deformity 113
aspiration
  causes 54
  recurrent in Parkinson's disease 53–6
ataxia
  hereditary 45–6
  management 46–8
  multiple sclerosis 45–48
  oscillopsia 47, 139
  patient assessment 45–6
  pharmaceutical therapy 47

attention
  components 32
  control 32
  retraining programmes 33
  strategies for improvement 33–4
attention deficit
  pharmacological management 32–4
  screening 32
attention-deficit hyperactivity disorder
    (ADHD) 33
autonomic dysreflexia 26–9
  bowel programme difficulties 129
  diagnosis 28
  differential diagnosis 28–9
  treatment 27–8
autonomic instability after brain
    injury 26–9
  diagnosis 28
autonomic neuropathy
  Charcot arthropathy 79
  hypotonic bladder 124–5
  persistent 119
Ayurvedic medicine 108

backward digit span 32, 40
baclofen 115
  intrathecal pump 116
  spastic paraplegia 113
  spasticity management 116
balance 148, 149
basilar artery thrombosis 29
behaviour, frontal lobe function testing 40
behavioural interventions, wandering patient 84
benzodiazepines 14
beta blockers in autonomic dysreflexia 27–8
bisphosphonates 63
  complex regional pain syndrome 96
  heterotopic ossification 68
bladder
  hypotonic 124–5
  intermittent catheterisation 124–5
  neuroanatomy 123–4
  sphincters 123–4
bladder outlet tightness 124–5
blindness
  denial 141
  see also cortical blindness
blood pressure dysregulation 27
bone fractures
  complex regional pain syndrome 94–5
  low impact 62, 63

bone mass
  assessment 62
  T and Z scores *62*
bone scintigraphy 95–6
botulinum toxin
  detrusor muscle injection 124
  detrusor sphincter dyssynergia 125
  equino varus deformity 112
  external urethral sphincter injection 124–5
  intravesical for neuropathic bladder 123–5
  nystagmus treatment 47
  oscillopsia treatment 47
  pontine myelinolysis 36
bowel
  dysfunction in spinal injury 126–9
  management following spinal injury 126–9
bowel programme 128
  difficulties 129
brachial neuritis *see* neuralgic amyotrophy
Braden scores, pressure sores risk assessment 64
bradykinesia, Huntington's disease 49
brain
  diffuse damage 135
  language function control 131
  localised damage 135–6
  visual cortex 140
brain injury
  aggression 41–3
  agitation following herpes simplex
      encephalitis 15–16
  anxiety following 20–3
  attention deficit 32–4
  autonomic instability 26–9
  ethnic minorities 85–7
  frontal lobe function assessment 37–40
  heterotopic ossification risk 67–8
  hormonal response 17
  hypopituitarism 17–20
  locked-in syndrome 29–31
  long-term prognosis 11
  medical issues 11
  mild 11
  patient needs 4
  pontine myelinolysis 34–7
  post-traumatic seizures 12–14
  severe 11, 12
  traumatic 11, 135
    cortical blindness 140–1
  vocational rehabilitation 149–51
  wandering patient 83–5
  see also post-traumatic amnesia (PTA)

Broca's area 131–2
  apraxia 133
bromocriptine
  attention deficit 34
  visual spatial neglect 144

calcium channel antagonists 24
calcium levels in immobility 61, 63
Campylobacter jejuni 117
cannabinoids, synthetic 94
capacity of patient 83–4
capsulitis, adhesive of shoulder 98
carbamazepine 13
  ataxia 47
  central pain syndrome 93
  herpes simplex encephalitis 16
cardiac complications of Duchenne muscular
      dystrophy 53
cardiovascular system, aerobic exercise 147
catastrophic cognition 22
cauda equina
  hypotonic bladder 124–5
  spinal injury 127
causalgia *see* complex regional pain syndrome
central pain syndrome 91–4
  neurosurgical procedures 94
  pharmaceutical management 92–3
  stroke 92–3
cerebral ischaemia, secondary 24
cerebral palsy
  foot drop 113
  patient needs 4
  scoliosis 71, 72
cerebrospinal fluid
  external lumbar drainage 25
  infusion test 25, 26
Charcot arthropathy 78–81
  amputation 80–1
  autonomic neuropathy 79
  infection 79–80
  management 79–81
  orthotics 80
  pathophysiology 79
  podiatry 80
  prostheses 81
  signs 79
Charcot retaining orthotic walker (CROW) 80
children
  chronic fatigue syndrome 90
  cortical blindness 141
  cortical visual impairment 140

chlorpromazine 49
cholecystitis in spinal injury 126–7
chorea, Huntington's disease 49
chronic fatigue syndrome 4
    children 90
    cognitive–behavioural therapy 89–90
    diagnosis 88, *88*
    differential diagnosis *89*
    Fukuda diagnostic criteria *88*
    graded exercise 88–9
    management 89–90
    physiotherapy 88–9
    rehabilitation team 89–90
    service provision 87–90
    severe disease 90
    support groups 89
chronic neurological disabilities 7
ciliac ganglia 127
citalopram 22
clobazam 14
clonazepam 47
clonidine, autonomic dysreflexia 27–8
Cobb angle 72
cognition, generalised deficits 135
cognitive–behavioural therapy 22
    chronic fatigue syndrome 89–90
    conversion syndrome *103*
    somatisation 106
cognitive estimates test 40
cognitive impairment
    cortical blindness 142
    diffuse brain damage 135
    frontal lobe dysfunction 37–8, *38*
    Huntington's disease 50
    localised brain damage 135–6
    mild brain injury 11
    pontine myelinolysis 36–7
    primary diffuse 135
    screening 39, *39*
    stroke 135–136
cognitive rehabilitation 135, 150
colostomy 129
coma, locked-in syndrome differential
        diagnosis 29, *30*
communication
    disabilities 130
    expressive aphasia 130–3
    hypokinetic dysarthria 136–8
    jargon aphasia 134–6
    language barriers in ethnic minorities 87
    pure disorders 135

strategies in aggression 42
communication aids
    locked-in syndrome 31
    non-fluent aphasia 132–3
complementary and alternative
        medicine 107–9
    classification *109*
    evidence of benefits 108
    placebo effect 108
    therapists 108
    use in rehabilitation 108–9
complex regional pain syndrome 94–7
    analgesia 96
    classification 95
    complications 96
    definition *95*
    diagnosis 95–6
    differential diagnosis *96*
    invasive techniques 96–7
    management 96–7
comprehension
    fluent aphasia 136
    mild aphasia 136
computer–brain interface 31
conduction aphasia 134–5
confusion 135
    cortical blindness 140
    pontine myelinolysis 35
constipation
    immobile neurological patients 127–8
    management *128*
constraint-induced therapy 145
consultation 3–5
conversion syndrome 4, 101–4
    assessment 102
    cognitive–behavioural therapy *103*
    diagnosis 102
    equipment 104
    management 102–4
    mobility aids 104
    psychological assessment 104
    secondary gains 104
coordination impairment 150
coronary angiography 140–1
cortical blindness 139–42
    causes 140–1
    children 141
    complete 140–2
    elderly patients 141
    management 141–2
    presentation 141

prognosis 142
  sleep disturbance 142
cortical visual impairment 140
cranial nerve paralysis 119
crystal therapies 107–8

dantrolene *115*
  spastic paraplegia 113
deep brain stimulation *48*
  ataxia 47–8
  central pain syndrome 94
de-escalation strategies 42
dehydration
  seizure trigger 13
  swallowing difficulties 54–5
dementia
  frontal lobe dysfunction 37–8
  screening 39
demyelination 35
  pontine 35
depersonalisation 22, *23*
depression
  following head injury 21
  Huntington's disease 49
  see also antidepressants
derealisation 22, *23*
desmopressin, intranasal 18
detention of patients 83
detrusor muscle 123–4
  botulinum toxin injection 124
  contraction 124
  sacral root stimulator device 128–9
detrusor sphincter dyssynergia 125
  botulinum toxin injection 125
  diagnosis 125
  investigations 125
  urodynamic studies 125
diabetes mellitus 78–81
diabetic ulcers 80
diaphragm 117, 121
  paralysis 120–2
  weakness 121
diazepam 14, *115*
diet, constipation management 127–8
discharge of patients 8
  destination 8
disinhibition, frontal lobe
      dysfunction 40
disodium etidronate 68
distraction techniques 22
domiciliary visits 5

dorsal reticulospinal tract 114
driving
  assessment 152–4
  contraindications 152
  in-car evaluation 152
  instruction 153
  on-road assessment 154
  peripheral vision 153
  pre-drive component 152
  professional tuition 154
  seating 153
  simulation 153
  vehicle modifications 153
  visual acuity testing 153
dual energy X-ray absorptiometry
      62
  indications *63*
Duchenne muscular dystrophy 45
  adult services 51–3
  cardiac complications 53
  genetics 51
  nutritional disorders 51–2
  respiratory failure 52
  scoliosis 52
  ventilation 52
  wheelchairs 51
dysarthria 137
  types *137*
dysphagia/dystonia in Huntington's
      disease 49
dystrophin 51

eating disorders, pontine
      myelinolysis 36
Ehlers–Danlos syndrome 71–2
elderly patients
  balance 149
  cortical blindness 141
employment, return to 149–51
encephalitis 135
  see also herpes simplex encephalitis
encephalomalacia 15
energy 146–7
  concept 107–8
  pathways *147*
environmental interventions, wandering
      patient 84
epilepsy
  diagnosis 16
  specialist nurses 44–5
  see also antiepileptic drugs; seizures

equino varus deformity
  muscles *111*
  neuroprostheses 113
  spasticity 110–13
  surgical management 113
equipment
  conversion syndrome patients 104
  provision 8
ethical issues 82
ethnic minorities 85–7
  comorbidities 86
  family role 86, 87
  language barriers 87
  perceived attitudes 86
  rehabilitation goals 87
  social isolation 87
executive function, higher 32
exercise 146–9
  aerobic 147
  balance 148, 149
  duration 147–8
  flexibility 148–9
  frequency 147–8
  graded in chronic fatigue syndrome 88–9
  health benefits *148*
  intensity 147–8
  post polio syndrome 76
  strengthening 148
expressive aphasia 130–3
eye blink/movement impairment 119

family
  ethnic minorities 86, 87
  wandering patient *85*
feeding, swallowing disorders 54
follicle-stimulating hormone 17, 18, *19*
foot drop
  cerebral palsy 113
  spastic 110–13
foot ulcers, diabetic 80
fractures *see* bone fractures
Frontal Assessment Battery (FAB) 39
frontal lobe
  damage and aggression 41
  dysfunction 37–8
    complications *38*
  function assessment 37–40
  pathology 38
  screening tests *39*, 39–40
functional electrical stimulation
  painful shoulder 99–100

peroneal nerve 113
functional tasks, extensive practice 33

gabapentin *115*
  ataxia 47
  central pain syndrome 93
  nystagmus treatment 47
gait
  abnormalities in post polio syndrome
    76, 78
  analysis 70
  assessment 70
    equino varus deformity 111–12
  ataxia 46
gastrocnemius muscle *111*
gastrocolic reflex 127
  bowel programme 128
gastro-oesophageal reflux 126–7
gastrointestinal tract, neural
    control 127
gastrostomy, percutaneous
    endoscopic 54
general anxiety disorder 21, *22*
Glasgow Coma Scale (GCS) 11, 175
global ischaemia, acute 24
glycerine suppositories 128
goal setting 7, 8
GP referrals 4
ground reaction force 70
growth hormone (GH) 17, 18, *19*
  replacement 20
  stimulation test 18
growth hormone-releasing hormone
    (GHRH) 18
Guillain–Barré syndrome 57–8
  autonomic dysfunction 119
  bladder management 119
  cranial nerve paralysis 119
  eye blink impairment 119
  immobility 58
  joints range of movement 119
  management 118–19
  nerve conduction studies 119
  prognosis 119
  respiratory failure 118
  vascular changes 58–9
  ventilatory support 117–19

haemorrhoids 129
hamstring spasticity 73
hand function, ataxia 46

heart rate
  maximal 147–8
  resting 148
heel ulcers 65
hemispheric stimulation in spatial
        neglect 145
herpes simplex encephalitis
  agitation following 15–16
  antiepileptic drugs 16
  differential diagnosis 16
  jargon aphasia 134–6
  psychiatric problems 15–16
  seizures 16
  status epilepticus 16
herpes simplex virus (HSV) 15
heterotopic ossification 67–9
  diagnosis 68
  functional assessment 68
  joint deformities 68–9
  NSAIDs 69
  recurrence 69
  risk factors 67–8
home adaptation 8
home leave 7–8
homonymous hemianopia 143
huntingtin 50
Huntington's disease
  behavioural manifestations 49–50
  frontal lobe dysfunction 37–8
  pathology 50
  physical manifestations 49
  prevalence 48
  psychiatric manifestations 48–50
hydrocephalus
  after subarachnoid haemorrhage
        23–6
  normal pressure 25
  shunt insertion 25–6
  signs 25
hyperalgesia, complex regional pain
        syndrome 95
hypercalcaemia 63
hypercalciuria 61
hyper-reflexive bladder 124
hypoalbuminaemia, pressure sores 65
hypogastric nerve 127
hypokinetic dysarthria 136–8
  clinical presentation 137
  speech therapy 137–8
hyponatraemia, pontine myelinolysis 35
hypopituitarism 17–20

diagnosis 18, 19
dynamic tests 18, 19, 20
hormone replacement 19, 20

ileostomy 129
immobility
  constipation 127–8
  heterotopic ossification 67–9
  medical complications 57
  osteoporosis 61
  pressure sores 64–7
  stroke 61–2
  thromboembolism 57–64
  thromboprophylaxis 58, 59–64
impulsivity, frontal lobe
        dysfunction 40
independence 146
indometacin 69
infection
  Charcot arthropathy 79–80
  pressure sores 66
informal patients 83
insight lack, fluent aphasia 136
insulin tolerance test 18, 19, 20
interdisciplinary work 7
intermediate rehabilitation units
        (IRUs) 7
intermittent catheterisation 124–5
intracranial pressure in hydrocephalus 25
isoniazide 47

jargon aphasia 134–6
job coach 151
joints
  contractures in pontine myelinolysis 36
  deformities in heterotopic ossification 68–9
  range of movement 119, 148–9
  stability in ataxia 46–7

keratitis, exposure 119

lamotrigine 13
  central pain syndrome 92, 93
language
  barriers in ethnic minorities 87
  function control 131
  functions 134
laxatives 128
length of stay 7–8
letter fluency tests 39–40
Lewy body dementia 37–8

locked-in syndrome 29–31
  causes 30
  classification 30
  communication 30–1, *31*
  conscious state assessment *31*
  diagnosis 30
  differential diagnosis 29, *30*
  pontine myelinolysis 35
lower limb
  spasms 65
  see also foot drop; foot ulcers
lower motor neurone lesions
  bowel dysfunction 127, *128*
  neuropathic bladder 124
luteinizing hormone (LH) 17, 18, *19*

magnetic resonance imaging (MRI), complex
      regional pain syndrome 95–6
malnutrition, swallowing difficulties 54–5
management plan 4–5
mattresses, pressure-relieving 65
maximal heart rate 147–8
medial reticulospinal tract 114
medical stability 6
medically unexplained conditions 4, 101
  conversion syndrome 101–4
  somatisation in multiple sclerosis 104–6
medication administration with swallowing
      disorders 56
medico-legal issues 82
  restraint 84
  wandering patient 83–5
memory deficit with brain injury 32
Mental Health Act, wandering patient 84, *85*
mental health problems
  family history 22
  following head injury 21–3
meridians 107–8
methylphenidate 33–4
  neuroprotective action 33–4
midazolam 14
Mini Mental State Examination (MMSE) 37, 39
mobility aids, conversion syndrome 104
Mobility Centre Static Assessment Rig 153
modafinil 34
mood
  pain 91
  see also anxiety; depression
morphine sulphate 28
motor cortex stimulation 94
motor impairment 150

motor neurone disease 45
motor neurone lesions *see* lower motor neurone
      lesions; upper motor neurone lesions
movement disorders, Huntington's disease 49
multidisciplinary approach 7
  severe brain injury 11
multiple sclerosis 7
  ataxia 45–8
  central pain syndrome 93–4
  fatigue 93
  generalised severe spasticity 113–16
  patient needs 4
  physiotherapy 44
  somatisation 104–6
  steroid therapy 61–2
  synthetic cannabinoids 94
multisystem atrophy 37–8
Munchausen's syndrome 102
muscles
  pseudohypertrophy 51
  tone in ataxia 47
muscular dystrophy
  scoliosis 72
  see also Duchenne muscular dystrophy
mutism 130–1, *132*
myelinolysis, extrapontine 35
myositis ossificans *see* heterotopic ossification

naming tests 39–40
narcolepsy 33
neck muscle vibration 145
negative pressure therapy, pressure sores 66–7
neglect
  clinical tests *144*
  lateralisation 143
  unilateral 143
  see also visual spatial neglect
neoplasms, cortical blindness 140–1
nerve conduction studies, Guillain-Barré
      syndrome 119
neuralgic amyotrophy 120–2
  diaphragmatic paralysis 121
  electromyography 120
  management 120, 121–2
  nerve conduction studies 120
  prognosis 121
  vital capacity 121
neurological rehabilitation 4
neuropathic bladder
  causes 124
  intravesical botulinum toxin 123–5

neuroprostheses, equino varus deformity 113
nimodipine 24
nominal impairment 131–2, 135
non-steroidal anti-inflammatory drugs *see*
    NSAIDs
    central pain syndrome 92
    heterotopic ossification 69
nutrition, constipation management 127–8
nutritional disorders
    Duchenne muscular dystrophy 51–2
    pontine myelinolysis 36
    swallowing difficulties 54–5
nystagmus 47

obsessive–compulsive disorder *22*
    Huntington's disease 49
on-the-job training 151
orthotics 70
    Charcot arthropathy 80
    equino varus deformity 112
    post polio syndrome 76, *77*
    scoliosis
        management 72–4
        secondary 71–4
oscillopsia 47, 139
ossification, heterotopic 67–9
osteopenia *62*
    complex regional pain syndrome 95–6
osteoporosis 61
    bisphosphonates 63
    risk stratification 63
    screening 62–3
    spinal injury 62
    stroke 62
osteotomy, equino varus deformity 113

pain, chronic 91
    central pain syndrome 91–4
    complex regional pain syndrome 94–7
    mood 91
    prognosis 91
    severity 91
    shoulder pain following stroke 97–100
pamidronate 63
    complex regional pain syndrome 96
pancreatitis, spinal injury 126–7
panhypopituitarism 18
panic disorder 21, *22*
paracetamol 28
paraphasias 132
paraplegia, spastic 113

parapyramidal tracts 114
Parkinson's disease 7
    deep brain stimulation 47–8
    frontal lobe dysfunction 37–8
    hypokinetic dysarthria 136–8
    physiotherapy 44
    recurrent aspiration 53–6
    specialist nurses 44–5
Parsonage–Turner syndrome *see* neuralgic
    amyotrophy
patients
    capacity 83–4
    explanation of seizure triggers 13
    needs 4
    philosophy of rehabilitation 7
percutaneous endoscopic gastrostomy 54
peripheral nerve injuries 94–5
peripheral vision, driving assessment 153
peroneal nerve, functional electrical
    stimulation 113
phenol, intrathecal injections 115–16
phenytoin 13
    acute post-traumatic seizures 12
philosophy of rehabilitation 7
phrenic nerve 117
    pacing 121–2
physiotherapy
    ataxia 46
    chronic fatigue syndrome 88–9
    neuralgic amyotrophy 120
    progressive neurological disorders 44
    scoliosis 73
    spasticity management 110
pituitary function assessment *20*
placebo effect 108
podiatry, Charcot arthropathy 80
poliomyelitis 74–8
    epidemic 74–5, 118
pontine myelinolysis 34–7
    neurological recovery 36
    outcomes 35
    pathology 35
    presentation 35
post polio syndrome 74–8
    diagnostic criteria *75*
    exercise 76
    management 76–8
    orthotics 76, *77*
    pathology 75
    prevalence 75
    signs 75, 78

post-concussion syndrome 11, 21
post-traumatic amnesia (PTA) 11, 12, 37
   attention impairment 32
post-traumatic stress disorder (PTSD) 21, *22*
pressure sores 64–7
   debridement 66, *66*
   infection 66
   management 65–7
   necrotic tissue removal 66, *66*
   negative pressure therapy 66–67
   risk assessment 64, 65
   shearing force 64
   staging *65*
primidone 47
prism adaptation, spatial neglect 145
progressive neurological disorders
     44–5
   see also Duchenne muscular dystrophy;
     Huntington's disease; multiple
     sclerosis; Parkinson's disease
progressive supranuclear palsy 37–8
prolactin 17
propranolol 27–8
proprioception 148, 149
prostheses
   Charcot arthropathy 81
   neuroprostheses in equino varus deformity
     113
pseudobulbar palsy 35, 36
pseudo-seizures 4
psychiatric impairment, pontine myelinolysis
     36–7
psychosis, Huntington's disease 49
psychotherapy interventions 108
pudendal nerve 127

quadriparesis, pontine myelinolysis 35

re-attribution model in somatisation 106
reflex sympathetic dystrophy 94–5
reflexology 107–8
rehabilitation clinic 3
rehabilitation physicians 3–4
rehabilitation team 3–4
   chronic fatigue syndrome 89–90
   complementary and alternative medicine
     use 108–9
rehabilitation unit 6–8
ReiKi 107–8
relaxation techniques 22
renography, spinal cord injury 125

respiratory dysregulation 27
respiratory failure
   Duchenne muscular dystrophy 52
   Guillain–Barré syndrome 118
restraint of wandering patient 84
rhizotomy, surgical 115–16
rigidity of thinking 40
rotator cuff
   muscles *99*
   shoulder impingement syndrome 98

saccular aneurysms
   clipping 24
   endovascular coiling 24
   subarachnoid haemorrhage 24
sacral root stimulator device 128–9
scanning training, spatial neglect 144–5
scientific medicine 107
scoliosis
   acquired 72
   assessment 72, *73*
   causes *73*
   cerebral palsy 71, 72
   classification 71–2, *73*
   congenital 71–2
   Duchenne muscular dystrophy 52
   idiopathic 71–2
   management 72–4
   physiotherapy 73
   secondary 71–4
seating
   driving 153
   secondary scoliosis 73–4
seizures
   complex partial 13
   diagnosis 13
   driving contraindication 152
   generalised 13
   herpes simplex encephalitis 16
   methylphenidate therapy 33
   partial 14
   pontine myelinolysis 35
   post-traumatic 12–14
     acute 12
     late 13
   refractory 14
   simple partial 13
   triggers 13
selective serotonin reuptake inhibitors (SSRIs)
     22–3
semiskilled workers 150

sensory disability 139
  cortical blindness 139–42
  visual spatial neglect 142–5
seven subtraction tests 32
shearing force, pressure sores 64
shoulder
  adhesive capsulitis 98
  hemiplegia 98
  impingement syndrome 98
  muscle spasticity 98
  pain following stroke 97–100
  range of motion 98
  TENS 99–100
shoulder–hand syndrome see complex regional
    pain syndrome
shunts
  acute dysfunction 26
  infection 26
  insertion in hydrocephalus 25–6
  partial obstruction 26
  ventriculo-peritoneal 26
sigmoid colostomy 129
sitting, secondary scoliosis 73–4
sleep apnoea syndrome 117
sleep disturbance, cortical blindness 142
sleeping systems, secondary scoliosis 73
social isolation, ethnic minorities 87
sodium valproate 93
soleus muscle 111
somatisation
  cognitive–behavioural therapy 106
  comorbidity 106
  multiple sclerosis 104–6
  re-attribution model 106
  stress association 106
  symptoms 105, 106, 106
spasticity
  ataxia 47
  clinical problems 114
  equino varus deformity 110–13
  generalised severe 113–16
  hamstring muscles 73
  intrathecal baclofen pump 116
  intrathecal phenol injections 115–16
  management 110, 115
  painful shoulder 100
  physiotherapy 110
  pontine myelinolysis 36
  shoulder 98
  surgical rhizotomy 115–16
  upper motor neurone lesions 114

venous thromboembolism risk 59
spatial neglect 143
  clinical assessment 143–4
  clinical tests 144
  dopamine deficiency 144
  scanning training 144–5
  therapeutic strategies 144–5
  unilateral 144
  see also visual spatial neglect
specialist nurses 44–5
speech
  control 137
  process 138
speech therapy 137–8
sphincteric dysfunction 123–5
  neuropathic bladder 123–5
spina bifida, patient needs 4
spinal cord stimulation, central pain syndrome
    94
spinal deformity assessment 72
spinal dorsal root stimulator 96–7
spinal injury/spinal cord injury
  autonomic dysreflexia 27
  bowel management 126–9
  cauda equina 127
  central pain syndrome 93
  detrusor sphincter dyssynergia 125
  gastrointestinal disorders 126–7
  heterotopic ossification risk 67–8
  high cervical 117, 118
  immobility 58
  osteoporosis 62
  patient needs 4
  renography 125
  thromboprophylaxis 58
  venous thromboembolism risk 58
spinal muscle atrophy 72
spinothalamic tract lesions 92
Static Assessment Rig (Mobility Centre) 153
status epilepticus 16
steroid therapy, multiple sclerosis 61–2
stool propulsion 127
stress, somatisation association 106
stretching 148–9
stroke
  arm function loss 97–8
  central pain syndrome 92–3
  cognitive impairment 135–6
  cortical blindness 139–42, 140–1
  driving assessment 152–4
  exercise 146–9

stroke (*cont.*)
  expressive aphasia 130–3
  immobility 61–2
  localised brain damage 135–6
  osteoporosis 62
  shoulder pain 97–100
  sleep apnoea syndrome 117
  visual spatial neglect 142–5
stroke volume 148
subarachnoid haemorrhage 135
  complications 24
  hydrocephalus 23–6
  rebleeding 24
subcortical dementia 37–8
Sudeck syndrome *see* complex regional pain
    syndrome
superior mesenteric artery syndrome 126–7
superior mesenteric ganglia 127
support groups, chronic fatigue syndrome 89
supported employment 151
swallowing
  assessment 54, 56
  function 53–4
  impairment *55*
  problems 54
  safety strategies *55*
sympathetic block, complex regional pain
    syndrome 96–7

tap test 25, 26
temperature dysregulation 27
TENS (transcutaneous electrical nerve
    stimulation) 99–100
tetrabenazine 49
thermography, complex regional pain
    syndrome 95–6
thinking, rigidity 40
thromboembolism 57–64
thromboprophylaxis in immobile patients 58,
    59–64
thyroid-stimulating hormone (TSH) 17,
    18, *19*
tibialis anterior muscle 111
  equino varus deformity *111*, 112
  surgical transfer 113
tibialis posterior muscle 111
  equino varus deformity *111*, 112
  surgical transfer 113
tizanidine *115*
topiramate 93
transcortical aphasia, motor/sensory 132

transcutaneous electrical nerve stimulation *see*
    TENS
transit time studies 129
traumatic brain injury 135
  cortical blindness 140–1
  medical issues 11
treatment decisions, capacity of patient 83–4
tremor, intention 47
tricyclic antidepressants 92–3
  amitriptyline 92
trunk stability, ataxia 46–7

unskilled workers 150
upper limb
  TENS 99–100
  see also arm; shoulder
upper motor neurone lesions
  bowel dysfunction 127, *128*
  neuropathic bladder 124
  sacral root stimulator device 128–9
  spastic foot drop 111
  spasticity 114
upper motor neurones, parapyramidal
    tracts 114
urethral sphincter, external 123–4
  botulinum toxin injection 124–5
urine retention with overflow 124–5
urodynamic studies, detrusor sphincter
    dyssynergia 125

vagus nerve 127
valproate 13
vegetative state 30
  locked-in syndrome differential diagnosis
    29, *30*
vehicle modifications 153, 154
  remote key pad 153, 154
ventilation
  Duchenne muscular dystrophy 52
  non-invasive nocturnal 52
  positive pressure 118, 121–2
ventilatory support 117
  Guillain–Barré syndrome 117–19
vestibulospinal tract 114
video fluoroscopy, swallowing
    assessment 56
visual acuity testing 153
visual cortex 140
visual disturbance 47
visual field defects 143
  driving contraindication 152

visual hallucinations 140, 141
  cortical blindness 142
visual impairment 139
  cortical 140
visual rehabilitation programme 141–2
visual spatial neglect 34, 142–5
  clinical assessment 143–4
  clinical tests *144*
  dopamine deficiency 144
  scanning training 144–5
  stroke 142–5
  therapeutic strategies 144–5
  unilateral 144
visual stimulation, repetitive 141–2
vital capacity, neuralgic amyotrophy
  121
vocational guidance and
  counselling 151

vocational rehabilitation 149–51
  commencing 150–1
  prognostic indicators 150, *150*

wandering patient 83–85
  behavioural interventions 84
  emergency situations 83
  environmental interventions 84
  guidelines *85*
  restraint 84
Waterloo scores, pressure sore risk
  assessment 64
Wernicke's aphasia 134
Wernicke's area 131–2
Wernicke's encephalopathy 36–7
wheelchairs
  Duchenne muscular dystrophy 51
  spatial neglect 143